Preventing Physical and Emotional Abuse of Children

TREATMENT MANUAL FOR PRACTITIONERS
David H. Barlow, *Editor*

PREVENTING PHYSICAL AND EMOTIONAL
ABUSE OF CHILDREN
David A. Wolfe

SEXUAL DYSFUNCTION
A GUIDE FOR ASSESSMENT AND TREATMENT
John P. Wincze and Michael P. Carey

SEVERE BEHAVIOR PROBLEMS
A FUNCTIONAL COMMUNICATION TRAINING APPROACH
V. Mark Durand

DEPRESSION IN MARRIAGE
A MODEL FOR ETIOLOGY AND TREATMENT
Steven R. H. Beach, Evelyn E. Sandeen,
and K. Daniel O'Leary

TREATING ALCOHOL DEPENDENCE
A COPING SKILLS TRAINING GUIDE
Peter M. Monti, David B. Abrams,
Ronald M. Kadden, and Ned L. Cooney

SELF-MANAGEMENT FOR ADOLESCENTS
A SKILLS-TRAINING PROGRAM
MANAGING EVERYDAY PROBLEMS
Thomas A. Brigham

PSYCHOLOGICAL TREATMENT OF PANIC
David H. Barlow and Jerome A. Cerny

Preventing Physical and Emotional Abuse of Children

DAVID A. WOLFE
The University of Western Ontario
and The Institute for the Prevention of Child Abuse

Editor's Note by David H. Barlow

THE GUILFORD PRESS
New York   London

© 1991 The Guilford Press
A Division of Guilford Publications, Inc.
72 Spring Street, New York, N. Y. 10012

Printed in the United States of America

This book is printed on acid-free paper

Last digit is print number   9 8 7 6 5 4 3 2

Library of Congress Cataloging-in-Publication Data

Wolfe, David A.
  Preventing physical and emotional abuse of children /   David A.
Wolfe
    p.   cm. — (Treatment manuals for practitioners.)
  Includes bibliographical references and index.
  ISBN 0-89862-208-5 (hardcover).   ISBN 0-89862-219-0 (pbk.)
  1. Child abuse—Prevention. 2. Psychological child abuse—
Prevention. 3. Parent and child. I. Title. II. Series.
  [DNLM: 1. Child Abuse—prevention & control.   WA 320 W8554]
RC569.5.C55W64   1991
362.7'67—dc20
DNLM/DLC
for Library of Congress   91-24679
                                                                   CIP

To my wife, Barb, and my children, Alex and Amy,
for showing me the meaning of parenthood

About the Author

David A. Wolfe (Ph.D., 1980, University of South Florida) is Professor of Psychology and Psychiatry at the University of Western Ontario in London, Canada, and is Co-Director of Clinical Training. He is the Director of Research at the Institute for the Prevention of Child Abuse in Toronto, where he is involved in the development of policy and research aimed at the prevention of child maltreatment. Dr. Wolfe holds a Diplomate in Clinical Psychology from the American Board of Professional Psychology, and maintains a practice in child clinical psychology with the Children's Aid Society of London/Middlesex.

His research interests focus primarily on adjustment disorders among children from violent and abusive families, and the treatment and prevention of child abuse. He received the "Contribution to Knowledge Award" from the Ontario Psychological Fundation in 1989 for his work with children of battered women. His past and present editorial board memberships include *Child Abuse & Neglect, Journal of Consulting and Clinical Psychology, Journal of Family Violence, The Journal of Interpersonal Violence, Journal of Clinical Child Psychology,* and *The Journal of Child Sexual Abuse.* He is co-author of *The Child Management Program for Abusive Parents* (with K. Kaufman, J. Aragona, and J. Sandler); *Children of Battered Women* (with P. Jaffe and S. Wilson); and is author of *Child Abuse: Implications for Child Development and Psychopathology.* He lives in London, Ontario with his wife and two children.

Editor's Note

Few problems presenting to mental health professionals are as tragic and pathetic as child abuse, whether physical or emotional. In recent times our social service agencies and public policy makers have become very sensitive to the extent and pervasiveness of this problem. These individuals and organizations have taken every step possible to draw attention to abuse when it occurs and to prevent additional abuse from occurring. Most often children are removed from the abusing environment, a solution that everyone agrees may be necessary but unfortunate. To date, attempts by mental health professionals to intervene have most often focused on reducing the abusing behavior of the parents or caretakers as well as on eliminating problematic behavior in children that may cue the abuse.

Now David Wolfe presents an important new program, which is the culmination of years of work in this difficult area, and in an important advance, extends the program down to infants and toddlers. This program is designed to enhance the development of the child by recognizing early signs of potential abuse and intervening in such a way as to maximize positive interactions in the family. This very realistic, down-to-earth, and practical program concentrates on positive development, thereby avoiding the necessity of focusing on punitive measures that may be necessary when the problem is more advanced. I think that most professionals would agree with that this constitutes one of the most important advances in this area in recent times.

David H. Barlow
University of Albany,
State University of New York

Preface

The program structure and clinical procedures described in this volume grew out of 15 years of effort by my students, my colleagues, and myself to discover methods that would be of practical and realistic use in helping to combat violence toward children. We came to view this complex phenomenon not as a function of parental maladjustment alone, but also as a function of the many negative factors impinging on families and the inadequate assistance being offered to counterbalance these influences.

This book offers suggestions and programmatic methods for early intervention and treatment in families at clear risk of physical and/or emotional child abuse. It was written to assist experienced practitioners and students who come into contact with such families on a regular basis, whether they are referred by the school because of child behavior problems, referred by child protective services because of abuse reports, or self-referred because of conflict and disharmony. It is intended to offer more than particular techniques that will make an abusive family become nonabusive, by presenting an intervention philosophy based on the belief that strengthening the parent–child relationship is at the center of child abuse prevention. The methods and suggestions throughout the volume, therefore, represent directions for assisting such families in a manner that is most likely to lead over time to success.

Most forms of family violence toward children (i.e., physical abuse, exposure to wife assault, and psychological abuse), as well as child-rearing inadequacies (e.g., emotional and physical neglect), entail many of the actions and circumstances that are indicative of socialization failure. We have entered a time in which there is a re-emphasis on family integrity as opposed to out-of-home placements; in conjunction with this movement, social service and mental health professionals are looking for ways to offer assistance to multiproblem families that can eliminate or reduce the need for protective supervision. This has produced a critical need to discover and implement different ways of preventing socialization failure well in advance of the establishment of physically or emotionally abusive patterns of child rearing.

Efforts to treat offenders and victims of child abuse are still very much in a developing stage. Since the early 1960s, views on the primary causes of child abuse have expanded considerably; they have moved beyond blaming disturbed individuals or disturbing children to include the pervasive influences of socioeconomic disadvantage, cultural sanctioning of violence and corporal punishment, and the breakup of the nuclear family. Although all of these forces undoubtedly contribute to the problem, they are regrettably not likely to decline in the immediate future. To compensate for these debilitating factors, it is incumbent on mental health professionals to play a larger role in helping parents and children to establish more healthy, violence-free relationships.

The basis of the approach outlined in this volume is that child abuse prevention can be best achieved by maximizing the child's developmental abilities through child-centered activities involving parents. The developmental orientation underlying this intervention program implies something of a departure from most current efforts to treat child victims of maltreatment and to prevent its recurrence. First of all, practitioners are encouraged to direct intervention efforts more toward the strengthening of developmentally relevant tasks or skills that will bolster the parent–child relationship, in addition to addressing specific presenting complaints. Equally important is the implication, based on this orientation, that prevention and intervention efforts can be planned from an earlier point in time in such a way that undesirable (and potentially problematic) developmental deficits can be minimized. Rather than relying on aversive contingencies (i.e., detecting abuse and neglect, and imposing changes on the family), this strategy works on the principle of providing the least intrusive, earliest assistance possible. The focus thus shifts more toward promoting an optimal balance between the needs of the child and the abilities and resources of the family.

The recommended treatment practices outlined in this book reflect the view that protective factors can be built into the parent–child relationship, if this process is begun early in the formation of this relationship, in a manner that is maximally sensitive to each family's strengths and weaknesses. Thus, once parental expectations and treatment priorities have been identified, this treatment program begins with methods that promote sensitive and enjoyable parent–child interactions. By providing the opportunity and direction to allow parents and children to enjoy each other's company, we are setting the stage for a strong relationship that has a greater chance of surviving the more challenging aspects of child rearing and family stress.

The book deals as well with methods of teaching, discipline, and anger management—perhaps the "heart" of child abuse treatment endeavors to date. Whereas in the past such efforts have been initiated right from the beginning of the referral, the present volume reflects our more seasoned view that parents will be more effective and appropriate in their discipline once the parent–child relationship has been established on a firmer foundation. Nonphysical punishment methods, in particular, are not very effective at solving child-rearing problems unless coupled with effective attention, teaching methods, and emotional expression.

I wish to acknowledge the considerable support, both financial and professional, that was provided over the years in which this research and clinical program was developed. First and foremost, this program originated from the pioneering efforts of my research advisor, Dr. Jack Sandler, in the Department of Psychology at the University of South Florida, to whom I am grateful and indebted. Agencies and professionals in the London, Ontario, community deserve high recognition for their ongoing support in the operation of this program over the past decade. In particular, Mr. Terry Sullivan (previous executive director) and Mr. John Liston (executive director), as well as the staff of the Children's Aid Society of London/Middlesex County deserve ample recognition and praise for their commitment and assistance throughout the development and operation of this program.

Although I am sole author of this guide, I share this recognition with previous and current graduate students at the University of Western Ontario, who have also contributed immensely to the growth and development of the treatment methods described in this book. In alphabetical order, I wish to thank Patricia Bourdeau, Sue Bryant, Darlene Elliot-Faust, Catherine Koverola, Louise LaRose, Ian Manion, Jeff St. Pierre, Susan Wilson, and my very dedicated research assistant, Betty Edwards, for their hard work and caring input. Anne Krupka deserves special mention for her major contribution (presented in Chapter 5) of procedures developed specifically for assisting parents with infants and toddlers. Without these individuals, who mostly volunteered their time and energy in exchange for training and experience, this program could not have operated. With major gratitude, I also wish to acknowledge the Medical Research Council of Canada, which provided major portions of the funding for the research and clinical program presented herein.

Finally, I would like to express considerable appreciation to my wife, Barb Legate, who has contributed in untold ways to the practical aspects of the child care methods described in this book. I must also thank my son, Alex, and my daughter, Amy, who tested my theories (and patience) in many ways that led to more realistic child-rearing advice. Since their birth I humbly recognize that I am less of an "expert," and mostly just another parent.

D.A.W.
London, Ontario

Contents

Preventing Physical and Emotional Abuse of Children

1

Defining Physical and Emotional Abuse in the Context of Child-Rearing Practices

The relatively recent upsurge of interest in the prevention and treatment of child abuse is partially due to the fact that society's thinking on this topic has evolved considerably in recent decades. Although child abuse has always been present, and most likely was even more commonplace in previous generations than it is today (Radbill, 1968), maltreatment of children was seldom identified as such, because society was more tolerant and accepting of harsh forms of discipline and parents' right to use corporal punishment than we are today. Another reason why history has been tarnished by our culture's abuse of children is that children are unable to speak out on their own behalf. Thus, rules and laws governing the treatment and care of children have always been up to the discretion of adults. Not surprisingly, the abuse of children also exists because of the fact that children, by their very nature, require considerable control on the part of adults, many of whom are ill prepared for this vital and challenging role. Consequently, such control often takes the form of physical coercion, corporal punishment, and other methods of attempting to punish undesirable behavior.

If child abuse has existed in many different forms throughout history, why have efforts been made only recently to counteract this cultural pattern of mistreating or ignoring the needs of children? Like many other major social issues of this century (e.g., abuse of women, sexism, ageism, racial discrimination), child abuse became the focus of concern only after a number of "crises" were highlighted and counts were made of the casualties emerging from our existing values and child-rearing practices. The seriousness and repugnance of physical abuse of children were thrust upon us by widespread mass media attention to several highly publicized cases. During this upswing in public attention in the 1960s and 1970s, pictures and stories of severely injured and mistreated children were commonplace in news magazines and television news reports. The medical profession, to its credit, developed better ways to detect old or recent broken bones or unusual patterns of injury, drawing further attention to the plight of these children and the deviant behavior such abuse represents.

In this manner, the stage was set to draw public concern to this phenomenon and to root out the causes of and contributors to such behavior. The problem of abuse of children had been "discovered" (it was first widely defined and publicized in the scientific literature by the publication on the "battered child syndrome" by Kempe, Silverman, Steele, Droegenmueller, & Silver, 1962). Moreover, the public could easily identify the "wrongness" of such behavior, in that no one could reasonably argue that such injuries to children were not of concern. This identifiable "problem" stood in stark contrast to some of the other, less easily defined social issues of the day (e.g., the rights of women and minorities), which to some were less urgent and perhaps even undeserving of attention or change in social policy.

Yet, in much the same way as the other social movements originating in the 1960s met with a clash of resistance from the status quo, the child protection movement (so named on the basis of its primary objective) met with a backlash of criticism and disagreement as to the causes of this problem and, more to the point, whom to blame, punish, or rehabilitate (see, e.g., Gelles, 1973; Gil, 1970; Light, 1973). So that the problem would be identified and responded to by the public and by government agencies, the most severe and shocking aspects of physical abuse were dramatized and publicized. Thus, over the past three decades it was not uncommon for the media and professionals alike to present child abuse as an extremely deviant, malicious act that could only be committed by a disturbed individual

What Is Physical Abuse?

From early attempts to understand and define physical child abuse, a false dichotomy unwittingly emerged that has influenced how this problem has been viewed for some time. Child-abusive parents were identified and described as if they represented a distinct group of parents who committed such acts as a result of their extreme personality and situational failures (cf. reviews by Spinetta & Rigler, 1972; Wolfe, 1985). Such a differentiation between abusers and nonabusers was supported by the suspicion that child abusers were qualitatively and quantitatively *distinct* individuals from nonabusers, based on the fact that they had been found guilty (by court of law or child welfare professionals) of physically injuring or marking a child. Thus, professional and public opinion held onto the belief for some time that child abuse is an extremely bizarre and deviant act, set apart from the types of behaviors that "normal parents" may show toward their own children (see Magnuson, 1983, for examples of media descriptions of this issue).

From its beginnings in the 1960s, moreover, thinking and responding to the diverse problem of child abuse have often left both professionals and the public in a dilemma regarding aceptable versus unacceptable treatment of children by caregivers. Consequently, actions to counteract this problem have been taken in response to public sentiment, highly publicized cases, new legislation, and promising treatment methods. Over the past two decades, for example, legal definitions of child physical abuse have attempted to clarify the nature of the physical injuries that constitute abuse, specifying in greater detail the types of physical evidence that constitute abuse, and the behavioral signs that indicate an abused child (Besharov, 1985). In contrast to these developments, the research community has begun to move beyond the relatively narrow significance of physical injuries alone, to focus more on the pervasive and long-standing psychological and developmental consequences of inadequate (i.e., abusive, neglectful, inappropriate) child rearing (e.g., Cicchetti, 1989; McGee & Wolfe, 1991). Unintentionally, these different purposes for defining abuse and maltreatment (i.e., legal purposes vs. social science purposes) have contributed to greater confusion and contradiction of terms, especially in reference to treatment and prevention strategies. For example, the meaning of the term "prevention" in the legal context (i.e., protecting children from physical harm) is very different from the social science emphasis on building and strengthening appropriate child-rearing methods in order to enhance the parent–child relationship.

Unfortunately, the term "child abuse" continues for many to imply only the most visible, highly publicized assaults on children. As a result of such failure to define this phenomenon in relation to the full range of normal and abnormal child-rearing practices, many individuals may fail to recognize their own inappropriate child-rearing methods. A dichotomy that divides "abusers" and "nonabusers," or "abusive acts" and "nonabusive acts," may have a necessary role in defining the terms for (involuntary) social intervention; however, as we see throughout this book, it offers little benefit to treatment. In fact, such a false dichotomy contradicts the necessary wide-scale recognition of our cultural failures and harmful socialization practices with children, and impairs efforts at noncoercive prevention of such difficulties (Wolfe, 1990).

Presently, legal definitions exist in all states and provinces in North America for physical abuse; these provide at least a starting point for defining both the role and scope of prevention and intervention. Based on the Criminal Code of Canada, the Child and Family Services Act of Ontario (CFSA; 1984) is representative of most legal definitions of physical abuse: "The child has suffered physical harm, inflicted by the person having charge of the child or caused by that person's failure to care and provide for or supervise and protect the child adequately" (Section 37(2)(a)). Mandatory intervention by a child protective services agency can only occur when there are reasonable and probable grounds to suspect that disciplinary practices place the child in jeopardy (Section 37(2)). The CFSA, therefore, adds that "For purposes of Section 37(2)(a), there must be some 'measurable injury,' and acceptable corporal punishment is not abuse." Undeniably, the intent of such statutes is to clarify that parents have the right and responsibility to discipline their children without state or provincial interference, and that such interventions should occur only when highly inappropriate physical discipline is alleged to have occurred. (A practical interpretation of these intentions is provided below, following the discussion of emotional abuse.)

The definition and understanding of child abuse have continued to evolve since the initial recognition and widespread public awareness of the problem, over 25 years ago. Rather than attempting to identify the more extreme forms of abuse and treat those offenders, the current perspective on this problem views child abuse along a continuum ranging from normal and acceptable forms of parenting at one end, to more extreme and violent forms of child care at the other end (e.g., Cicchetti & Rizley, 1981; Burgess, 1979; Sameroff & Chandler, 1975; Wolfe, 1987). Such a continuum places this problem clearly within the context of socialization practices, rather than isolating it as deviant or criminal behavior. Directions for treatment and prevention are significantly advanced by such a perspective, because "child abuse" becomes less of the targeted treatment goal and more of a descriptive term that encompasses many of the more harmful and extreme forms of child rearing. Treatment objectives become considerably more definable and obtainable, because "treatment" can be defined in terms of what is best for the parent–child relationship.

What Is Emotional Abuse?

Recently, public and professional attention has been drawn to the even less visible, but perhaps more damaging, phenomenon of psychological or emotional abuse. There is a growing consensus among professionals that emotional abuse (or emotional maltreatment, in the more generic sense) is more prevalent than other forms of maltreatment, and is more destructive in its impact on development (Brassard, Germain, & Hart, 1987; Garbarino, Guttman, & Seeley, 1986; Rosenberg, 1987; McGee & Wolfe, 1991). However, prevalence estimates are currently very unreliable, given the problems associated with defining this nonphysical form of abuse.

Many researchers and practitioners have argued, quite convincingly, that a child's development and adjustment are affected by much more than the overt violence alone that historically has defined child abuse. The child is harmed as well by the accompanying (or independent) negative communications and emotional battery that result from constant scolding, criticism, and degradation in the child's everyday life. According to this argument, some children may be capable of adapting to or even accepting harsh and abusive physical actions from caregivers in the context of discipline. Historically, physical abuse has been considered wrong and harmful primarily because of the *physical* risk this poses to the victim. However, we have added to our understanding the recognition that physical injuries are not the only negative factors. Children are less successful in compensating for the absence of parental sensitivity, emotional responsiveness, or predictability, or for the presence of cruelty or exploitation; either of these sets of factors is generally defined as psychological abuse.

As a colleague and I have noted elsewhere (McGee & Wolfe, 1991), confusion over what constitutes "psychological abuse" can be reduced to two primary questions: First, what is meant by "psychological," and second, does the adjective "psychological" refer to parent behaviors or to child outcomes? A widely cited definition of psychological abuse or maltreatment was offered by Garbarino et al. (1986) and further clarified by Hart, Germain, and Brassard (1987):

> Psychological maltreatment of children and youth consists of acts of commission and omission which are judged on a basis of a combination of community standards and professional expertise to be psychologically damaging. Such acts are committed by individuals, singly or collectively, who by their characteristics (e.g., age, status, knowledge, organiza-

tional form) are in a position of differential power that renders a child vulnerable. Such acts damage immediately or ultimately the behavioral, cognitive, affective, or physical functioning of the child. Examples of psychological maltreatment include acts of rejecting, terrorizing, isolation, exploiting, and missocializing. (Hart et al., 1987, p. 6)

Although this concept is even more slippery to define than "physical abuse" for purposes of legal intervention, social policy, or treatment, the term clearly implies that much more is at stake than physical injuries alone in terms of what may define harsh parental treatment and its diverse impact on the child. Whereas in physical abuse the primary damage is considered the physical injuries to the child victim, psychological abuse inflicts injuries on such nonphysical (and often intangible) aspects of the individual as self-esteem, self-concept, and social competence (Garbarino et al., 1986).

With rare exception (e.g., Newfoundland, Alberta), there are few legally mandated definitions of emotional or psychological abuse of children that specify a threshold or criterion for state intervention. However, the degree of deviance that a given child must display in order to be considered in need of protection (with the nature of parental acts left unspecified) has been described in several legal references. According to the American Bar Association (Corson & Davidson, 1987), coercive intervention is warranted only when a child is already suffering serious emotional damage, as evidenced by severe anxiety, depression, withdrawal, or untoward aggressive behavior toward self or others, and the child's parents are unwilling to provide treatment for him. Similarly, the National Institute of Mental Health defines psychological abuse as "that which can be diagnosed in the presence of parental acts of omission or commission...when paired with the child's emotional, behavioral, and overall developmental deviations of sufficient degree as to suggest an imperative need for intervention for the child's safety and well-being" (Lauer, Lourie, Salus, & Broadhurst, 1979, p. 1).

Indisputably, physical abuse and emotional abuse can and often do exist concurrently, and at present we have insufficient knowledge to suggest which may be the more harmful. Previous definitions of these forms of maltreatment have relied on broad labels to categorize children and parents (e.g., "physically abused"). The point that must be derived from these recent attempts to clarify both concepts is that the labels "physical abuse" and "emotional abuse" do not indicate uniform, well-defined, or unique phenomena. These labels can obscure differences in the severity of abuse and ignore the co-occurrence of other forms of abusive actions (McGee & Wolfe, 1991). Their potential for misuse remains critical in defining the population of parents who may require state intervention, in particular. For the present purpose of defining those parents who may qualify for or need assistance with child rearing, however, the term "abuse" is used more or less generically to underscore the crucial emphasis on overall child-rearing practices.

What Are the Goals and Boundaries of Parental Discipline?

From a socialization perspective, child abuse can be viewed in terms of the extent to which parents use negative, inappropriate control strategies with their child, including psychological as well as physical strategies (Wolfe, 1987). Many of the different "types" of abuse (e.g., cruelty, denigration, physical assaults) often have one major thing in common: They signify the extremes to which a given parent may go in attempting to "discipline" his or her child, and the parent's lack of sensitivity to the child's limitations and needs.

Developmental researchers (e.g., Baumrind, 1971; Maccoby & Martin, 1983) have long argued that very dissimilar approaches to child rearing can emerge from the interaction of two fundamental dimensions of parenting: the degree of parental *demandingness* and the degree of parental *sensitivity.* Parents who are high on both dimensions are demanding of the child, while at the same time sensitive to the child's abilities and needs. Although this "parenting style" (described as "authoritative") is considered to be the most effective in terms of both discipline and enhancement of the parent–child relationship, all other combinations of these two dimensions result in greater or lesser degrees of parental ineffectiveness, harshness, or indifference to the child. For example, parents who are very demanding, yet fail to recognize a young child's limitations and needs, typify the pattern of many physically and emotionally abusive or harsh parents. In contrast, those who place very few demands or little structure on their children's behavior, while at the same time being unresponsive to their needs, exemplify the more neglectful, uninvolved style of parenting. These two dimensions of parenting, therefore, provide important reference points for establishing the goals and boundaries pertaining to parental discipline and child-rearing methods.

Physical discipline of children is a complex and contentious subject that has many implications for child abuse prevention. Some difficulty emerges in attempts to define the broad meaning of "child abuse," because our culture has long taken for granted that corporal punishment is a primary and necessary component of child discipline. Unfortunately, many parents are unfamiliar with alternative methods of punishment, and may fail to realize that discipline involves considerably more effort and planning than does punishment alone. Moreover, child-rearing practices in North America have clearly been changing over the past 50 years or so. Parents are expected to appreciate their child's developmental limitations and progress, and to move away from disciplinary methods that emphasize control toward ones that encourage the child's emerging independence and self-control. Despite these trends, however, major differences remain between various segments of the population concerning the extent of physical "abuse" of children that is deemed appropriate and acceptable (Gil, 1970).

What are some of the arguments against physical punishment as a disciplinary method? Campbell (1989) points out that one major criticism of physical punishment is that it does not facilitate learning; rather, punishment teaches children what *not* to do, and by itself would fail to teach children what is expected of them. "Discipline," on the other hand, refers to methods that permit the child to reduce undesirable behavior while learning alternative, appropriate actions.

In addition, physical punishment requires certain conditions for it to be effective—the very conditions that can easily get out

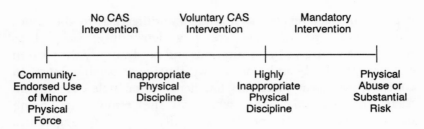

| No CAS | Voluntary CAS | Mandatory |
| Intervention | Intervention | Intervention |

| Community-
Endorsed Use
of Minor
Physical
Force | Inappropriate
Physical
Discipline | Highly
Inappropriate
Physical
Discipline | Physical
Abuse or
Substantial
Risk |

FIGURE 1.1. Continuum of physical discipline. From *Position Paper on Physical Discipline* by the Children's Aid Society of the Regional Municipality of Peel [Ontario], 1988, unpublished manuscript. Reprinted by permission of the Society.

of control and lead to abuse. As Campbell (1989) notes, in order for physical punishment to be an effective learning tool to any degree, it must be administered in such a fashion that the pain is as harsh or intense as possible, the pain is felt repeatedly, and no delay occurs between the occurrence of the behavior and the infliction of punishment. The delivery of physical punishment requires, almost by definition, that the adult become very emotionally aroused and angry. Such conditions further the potential for abuse because they decrease the adult's ability to plan and execute a decision rationally, and increase the risk of venting frustrations on the child that are unrelated to the child's problem behavior. Simply stated, the use of physical punishment increases the risk of physical and psychological harm to the child, primarily as a result of the manner in which it must be delivered; moreover, the other negative child-rearing methods that accompany its use (i.e., various degrees of emotional abuse) render this method questionable at best.

Legal definitions of physical abuse currently rest on the notion of "appropriate" versus "inappropriate" physical discipline of children. Unfortunately, however, no consensus exists on this subject that is easily translated into community standards or guidelines for families. In an attempt to clarify this issue, the Children's Aid Society (CAS) of the region of Peel, Ontario (a mandated child protection agency) provides a continuum model of physical discipline that is useful to our formulation of prevention and intervention goals. At one end are those physical discipline methods that have wide community acceptance, and at the other end are those methods defined as physical abuse by the provincial statute. Figure 1.1 illustrates the CAS continuum and the concerns or actions that various types of discipline might initiate.

In helping to establish the boundaries of physical discipline, the CAS offers the following operationalizations of the first three terms used in Figure 1.1:

(i) *Community-Endorsed Use of Minor Physical Force.* The Society accepts that there are instances when the use of minor physical force, such as spanking over clothes or pulling on a child's coat collar, may be perceived as necessary—for example, with very young children who, lacking an awareness of danger, thrust themselves into dangerous situations. For a very young child, about to run across a busy street, or about to put his hand on a hot object, the parent must act quickly to protect the child—and this could mean a sudden pulling at the child's clothing, or a gentle spanking on the rear, over the child's clothing, or a gentle tapping on the child's hand—and these methods are used to teach the child about potential dangers, to get the child's attention, and to divert him from possible harm. The Society would not have concerns with these parental actions, and would have neither a right nor an intent to intervene.

(ii) *Inappropriate Physical Discipline.* When parents move beyond the level of occasional and mild use of physical discipline, there is heightened cause for concern. A pattern of frequent use of physical discipline, such as spankings or hand slapping or jerking the child by the arm, may not cause physical injury, but are seen by child welfare professionals as inappropriate parenting methods. We believe that all professionals who work with children and families have a responsibility to discuss such practices with parents in an attempt to influence the parents to avail themselves of services which will help them to learn more effective methods of disciplining their children. We do not consider the

pervasive community problem of inappropriate child-
rearing practices to be the exclusive responsibility of
the Children's Aid Society. We do, however, recognize
our shared responsibility with all other child welfare
professionals in meeting this community service need.
The Society comes in contact with many families and
children in the course of discharging its child protec-
tions responsibilities. The Society undertakes to provide education and counselling in the area of alternatives to physical punishment for families receiving
services from the Society.

(iii) *Highly Inappropriate Physical Discipline.* Peel CAS takes
the position that there are reasonable grounds for sus-
pecting that a child may be in need of protection when
parents use highly inappropriate physical discipline. It
is incumbent upon professionals who become aware of
such child-rearing practices to discuss with the Children's Aid Society, and to develop jointly a plan of
intervention with these families. The factors to be considered in evaluating whether the use of corporal punishment is highly inappropriate are:

(a) *Method.* No parent or caregiver should use a weapon
on any part of the child's body. Belts, sticks, electrical
cords, hairbrushes, wooden spoons or other utensils are
examples of "weapons." Obviously, the use of any
weapon to discipline is of concern, given the potential
for injury. Similarly, the punching, kicking, or slapping of a child by an adult is a cause for concern. The
specific circumstances need to be evaluated in order to
determine the level of concern.

(b) *Severity.* The severity or harshness of the physical
discipline must be taken into consideration in determining the seriousness of the allegation. The amount of
force and the part of the child's body that is struck
determine the severity. Physical discipline may be considered severe and highly inappropriate in some situations when minimal force is applied. For example,
hitting or slapping a child about the head, face, or neck
area is considered a severe action and of great concern,
regardless of the force applied, because of the potential
for physical harm.

(c) *Frequency*. A pattern of use of physical discipline increases our concern for the well-being of the child, given the increased potential for injury, and for long-term psychological problems for the child.

(d) *Age*. The potential for injury from physical discipline to young children is particularly high. Infants, toddlers, or preschoolers are especially vulnerable. Medical evidence is clear, for example, that serious internal injuries can result from shaking, dragging, or throwing an infant.

(e) *Context*. The family circumstances that are related to use of physical discipline must be examined. If other indicators of abuse exist—for example, social or emotional problems of parents—the use of corporal punishment is of more concern because of the increased risk of abuse. (CAS, 1988, pp. 5–8; reprinted by permission of CAS)

TABLE 1.1. Continuum of Parental Emotional Sensitivity and Expression

Child-centered
- Provides a variety of sensory stimulation and positive emotional expressions; engages in highly competent, child-centered interactions
- Occasionally scolds, criticizes, interrupts child activity; emotional delivery and tone sometimes harsh

Borderline
- Shows rigid emotional expression and inflexibility in responding to child; uses verbal and nonverbal pressure to achieve unrealistic expectations
- Frequently uses verbal and nonverbal coercive methods and minimizes child's competence; is insensitive to child's needs; makes unfair comparisons and takes advantage of child's dependency.

Inappropriate/abusive
- Denigrates, insults child; expresses conditional love and ambivalent feelings toward child
- Emotionally or physically rejects child's attention; uses cruel and harsh control methods; shows no sensitivity to child's needs; intentionally seeks out ways to frighten, threaten, or provoke child; responds unpredictably with emotional discharge

14

A similar continuum describing the boundaries of *nonphysical* (i.e., emotional and nonverbal) discipline and child care can be described, although this area is less developed and specific than that for physical abuse. In Table 1.1, this continuum is extended in both the positive and negative directions, to emphasize the notion that emotional abuse represents one extreme of the dimension of parental sensitivity–insensitivity.

At the positive end of this continuum are the types of parental behaviors known to be highly favorable to child development. Highly competent parents provide a selective variety of stimulation to their children, and make every effort to match their demands and expectations to the needs and abilities of each child. Of course, parents are only human, and so the continuum recognizes that many parents will on occasion scold, criticize, or even show insensitivity to a child's state of need (in fact, discipline often requires such firm control, with accompanying verbal statements and affect).

The borderline and abusive actions represented along this continuum, however, represent greater and greater degrees of irresponsible and harmful child care. It is felt that parents who show these actions toward their children to any measurable extent could benefit from instruction and assistance in effective child care methods. Moreover, one could easily argue that those parents who engage in any of the actions falling at the abusive end of the continuum of emotional sensitivity and expression should receive the same degree of supervision and official intervention that is mandated for physical abuse.

The definition of emotional abuse, therefore, must take into account the wide variability in child-rearing practices, ranging from desirable to borderline to clearly inappropriate. This approach is similar to the CAS guidelines for physical discipline, in that it assumes no "cutoff" point at which a parent's action becomes abusive. Rather, it demonstrates the position that some actions are more desirable and appropriate than others, and that those parental behaviors falling at the negative end of the continuum pose considerable harm to the child's psychological development. For purposes of intervention, the continuum offers a beginning point for the specification of therapeutic goals beyond merely the cessation of physically inappropriate or abusive actions; it stresses that these goals should include desirable emotional expression and sensitivity.

From the discussion above, it is clear that parental discipline implies considerably more than one's choice of punishment procedure. Disciplining children requires an understanding of their developmental abilities and limitations, their particular style of behavior, expectations for change that are concordant with their maturity, and a great deal of time and patience.

No particular "technique" can provide the answer to the question of how to discipline, because every child and every situation offer new challenges. This fact of life often conflicts with disciplinary strategies that rely on aversive procedures (whether physical or emotional), for two principal reasons. First, those who employ aversive procedures may fail to balance their use of such procedures with positive disciplinary strategies that promote learning (e.g., providing the child with alternative choices; rewarding compliance and desirable behavior frequently). Also, the nature of aversive control methods affords the user with a simple and deceptively effective disciplinary armory to fit any need: The user can simply adjust the severity of the physical or emotional pain to match the severity of the child's misbehavior. Because the user is often reinforced in the short term by the quick cessation of the child's annoying behavior, he or she continues to adhere steadfastly to such aversive methods. However, the longer-term effects of overly harsh, punitive methods on children's behavior often go unrecognized; that is, children habituate to the initial level of pain, thereby requiring more intense and frequent delivery of punishment to have the desired effect on behavior. Moreover, harsh punishment teaches children the importance of not getting caught, thus serving to sharpen their skills at deception and avoidance (Wolfe, Kaufman, Aragona, & Sandler, 1981).

In view of these concerns about the goals and boundaries of disciplinary methods, we need to consider that emotional and physical forms of child abuse do not simply involve parental *misdeeds* (i.e., excessive and inappropriate behavior toward the child). Abuse also involves the *absence* of appropriate methods of child stimulation, sensitivity, and direction. Attempts at the prevention of child abuse, therefore, can be made considerably more efficacious if efforts are made to assist family members in the use of more appropriate and beneficial child care techniques. Such techniques and methods for enhancing the parent–child relationship are the true targets of child abuse treatment efforts.

A Sociodemographic Profile of Abusive Families

An understanding of the sociodemographic background from which most at-risk families may originate is helpful in planning intervention. In recent years, epidemiological studies of child abuse have provided a useful descriptive profile of this phenomenon, and have illuminated many of the cultural forces that surround childrearing methods and that contribute directly to parental aggression. Such epidemiologic variables associated with abuse, such as low income, unemployment, and family instability, provide important "markers" for identifying high-risk groups in society, thus allowing for subsequent investigations into the causal mechanisms connecting these variables to abusive parenting. Although such sociodemographic variables are clearly associated with elevated reports of child abuse, it is important to caution that their role may be an *indirect*, rather than a causal, influence on such reports. Many individuals who are disadvantaged do not exhibit any major parenting problems, and thus it is suspected that abuse may be the result of an *interaction* between such negative factors and the individual's (or family's) coping resources (e.g., Ammerman, 1990; Belsky, 1980; Starr, 1979; Wolfe, 1987).

Child Victims

Findings from the U.S. National Study on the Incidence and Severity of Child Abuse and Neglect (National Center on Child Abuse and Neglect [NCCAN], 1981, 1988) and from the U.S. National Study on Child Neglect and Abuse Reporting (American Humane Association [AHA], 1984) indicate that the average child victim of "abuse" (which covers, in this large data base, all forms of maltreatment) is relatively young (average age of 7.4 years), in comparison to the average age of all children in the United States (9.6 years). Interestingly, the highest rates of physical *injury* are found among the two extreme age groups: infants and toddlers on the one hand, and adolescents on the other. This latter finding may seem surprising at first, in light of the public image of this problem as centering primarily on very small children, but it makes sense in consideration of the extent of parent–child conflict that often emerges during these two developmental periods.

Little difference has been detected in terms of the child victims' sex, with boys and girls being reported as abused at approximately the same rate. It has also been shown by these national studies that the percentages of white and black children are largely representative of the U.S. population at large. However, reports made on black children are more likely to involve neglect, whereas white families have been characterized by more physical abuse or combined abuse and neglect.

Abusive Parents and the Family Context

To turn to information regarding caregivers who have been officially documented as abusive, it has been found that natural parents are the offenders in the majority of physical abuse reports. Moreover, the data tell us that abusive parents often began their families at a younger age than did other families in the population, with many being in their teens at the birth of their first child (AHA, 1984; NCCAN, 1981). Such findings underscore the importance of early parenting programs and guidance for young parents.

Although more female than male caregivers are reported for child maltreatment (60.8% female, 39.2% male), this finding must be qualified by the fact that child-rearing responsibilities fall predominantly on women, and by the fact that this figure represents all forms of maltreatment (not just physical abuse). In addition, the finding of more female than male offenders does not adequately reflect the seriousness of the reports. In terms of injuries to the child, male offenders are associated with more *major and minor physical injury*; males are also responsible for the vast majority of sexual abuse. In contrast, females are significantly more likely than males to be reported for child neglect. This latter finding of more neglect among females may be linked to the greater likelihood of adverse socioeconomic factors in female-headed households.

Finally, it is important to consider the socioconomic background factors associated with many of those families that have been reported for child abuse. National incidence data show that child maltreatment (i.e., all forms of maltreatment, including physical abuse) occurs disproportionately more often among economically and socially disadvantaged families (AHA, 1984; NCCAN, 1981, 1988). When compared to all U.S. children, for example, maltreated children are twice as likely to live in a single-parent, female-headed household; are four times as likely to be supported by public assistance; and are affected by numerous stress factors that impinge upon family functioning (such as health problems, alcohol abuse, and wife battering).

Although it is clear that a relationship exists between lower socioeconomic status and child maltreatment, it is also important to recognize that maltreatment does occur to varying degrees at all socioeconomic levels. When physical abuse is compared to neglect, however, some of the differences in terms of socioconomic background become more evident. For example, neglectful families are considerably below the national average on several socioeconomic indicators (47.6% of the neglectful families vs. 17.3% of all U.S. families are receiving public assistance; 44.1% vs. 6.5% are unemployed), but abusive families are closer to the U.S. average on these measures.

These socioeconomic differences between abusive and neglectful families notwithstanding, it is important to consider the relative importance of such contextual factors when planning intervention for at-risk families, especially those factors that may curtail the impact of treatment the most (e.g., insufficient housing or income; poor medical care, etc.). Clearly, the relative importance of assisting the family through social support, financial support, child management, or any other single or combined means must be ascertained early in the course of any intervention.

2

Causes and Consequences of Abusive Behavior

Treatment directions for child abuse have paralleled the predominant theoretical frameworks used to explain this phenomenon over the past three decades. As in most other areas of treatment of psychopathology, the development of treatment strategies for child abuse has involved a long process of trial and error, in which currently popular ideas have been heralded as the "necessary ingredients" for successful treatment outcome, only to be usurped by more popular methods or to fade because of disappointing results.

As an introduction to the theory behind the ideas and procedures described in this book, an overview of the early conceptualizations of child-abusive behavior is provided. Selected treatment approaches derived from these emerging explanations are also described, because they have formed the basis for important developments in intervention strategies. I then review some of the effects that parental abuse may have on children's development, prior to presenting an intervention model linked to critical transition periods for family members.

Explanations for Abusive Behavior

Psychopathology of the Parents

One of the first explanations for child abuse to be widely espoused by professionals following the recognition of the problem in the early 1960s was spawned by the early medical view of this phenomenon. Because, for the most part, pediatricians and other medical personnel were the ones who brought the problem of abuse to worldwide attention, attempts to explain this phenomenon were couched predominantly in terms of the individual psychopathology of the offender. Child abuse was a deviant act; therefore, it was reasoned that the perpetrators of such acts were themselves deviant (Spinetta & Rigler, 1972). The search began for the psychiatric symptoms or psychopathological processes that were responsible for such inhumane behavior by parents toward their offspring.

A number of important diagnostic signs of abuse were identified on the basis of this psychopathology viewpoint, as reported in early clinical studies. As summarized in Table 2.1, the most predominant behavioral characteristics of abusive parents included chronic, multisituational aggressive behavior, isolation from family and friends, rigid and domineering interpersonal style, impulsivity, and/or problems rooted in marital difficulties. At an emotional or cognitive level, such parents were described as being emotionally immature (e.g., they were thought to expect their children to "care" for them); as showing low frustration tolerance (especially for child-related stress); as having difficulties expressing anger appropriately, to have high expectations for their children (with little regard for the children's needs and abilities); and as possessing deep-seated problems in self-esteem and/or personality adjustment that were related to problems in their families of origin (in particular, their own poor treatment). Unfortunately, these initial descriptive findings remained largely speculative, due to the poor methodological underpinnings of research in this area at the time (methodology, incidentally, remains a challenging problem; see Mash & Wolfe, 1991).

Attempts to define child abuse during this period focused predominantly on the importance of tangible, physical injuries to

TABLE 2.1. Psychological Characteristics of Abusive Parents Reported in Early Clinical Studies

I. *Behavioral Dimension*
- Chronically aggressive (9)
- Isolated from family and friends (11)
- Rigid and domineering (9, 11)
- Impulsive (3, 4, 7, 11, 12)
- Experiencing marital difficulties (7)

II. *Cognitive–Emotional Dimension*
- Emotional immaturity (11)
- Low frustration tolerance (4, 7, 11, 12)
- Difficulty expressing anger (4, 7, 11, 12)
- Role reversal; looks to child to gratify own needs (2, 4, 5, 6, 10)
- Deficits in self-esteem (1, 2, 5)
- Inability to empathize with children (6, 8)
- High expectations of child; disregard for child's needs and abilities (6, 8, 10)
- Defends "right" to use physical punishment (12)
- Deep resentment toward own parents for failing to satisfy dependency needs.

Note. The following references to original studies are representative and not exhaustive. Most findings involved inferences drawn from clinical samples, without control group comparisons: (1) Bell (1973); (2) Blumberg (1974); (3) Elmer (1963); (4) Green (1976); (5) Green et al. (1974); (6) Helfer (1973); (7) Kempe et al. (1962); (8) Melnick & Hurley (1969); (9) Merrill (1962); (10) Morris & Gould (1963); (11) Steele & Pollock (1968); (12) Wasserman (1967). Also, see reviews by Green (1978); Kelly (1983); Parke & Collmer (1975); and Spinetta & Rigler (1972). The table is from *Child Abuse: Implications for Child Development and Psychopathology* (p. 71) by D. A. Wolfe, 1987, Newbury Park, CA: Sage. Copyright 1987 by Sage Publications. Reprinted by permission of the publisher.

the child that could not be explained on the basis of accidental or unpreventable parental actions (described often as "acts of commission or omission"; Kempe & Helfer, 1972). That is, an act was considered to be abusive if the parent did something that could lead to harm or physical consequences to the child, or the parent failed to perform some caregiving behavior that also led to harm or jeopardy to the child. In keeping with the psychopathology viewpoint, the focus of this definition was predominantly on the parent's behavior or deviancy, as well as visible evidence of the consequences of such behavior to the child. Accordingly, the more extreme cases of harsh or inappropriate parental behavior were more likely to be identified as abusive.

As noted in Chapter 1, such a definitional approach unfortunately resulted in a dichotomy between those parents who were considered to be "abusers" and those parents who were not, which was sometimes an arbitrary division that did little to advance assistance to families or public recognition of the problem. The hallmark of such a definition was the presence of unexplained or nonaccidental injuries to the child, which are often difficult to confirm. Paradoxically, a parent could be considered to have committed an "abusive act" if the injuries to the child were decreed as unexplained or deemed nonaccidental; or, conversely, a parent could be labeled as "abusive" if a child had only minor or equivocal physical injuries, given that the parent was decreed to be psychiatrically disturbed. Thus, the problem of (physical) child abuse produced considerable definitional ambiguity and confusion; this confusion tended to lead to criminalization of the behavior, rather than to efforts to prevent such serious parent–child problems in the least intrusive manner.

In conjunction with this early view, public awareness campaigns stressed the physical consequences to the child victims and the horrific experiences that some children may be put through at the hands of their parents. Such campaigns further reinforced the notion that disturbed and deviant individuals commit such acts, and therefore that society should support efforts to detect such individuals and limit their parental rights. In a manner of speaking, child abuse was seen as the symptom of a broader disorder, and its treatment followed accordingly (i.e., identification of the disorder, with individual treatment prescribed).

This psychopathology-based view of child abuse led to treatment efforts directed primarily at individual parents. Because it was assumed that child abuse was the result of parental personality disturbance, most treatment focused on parents' insight into their own past experiences, which often included abuse by their own caregivers. In addition, treatment efforts explored the use of home monitoring or counseling, supplying paraprofessionals to assist in reducing the amount of chaos or stress existing in the family (see examples of such efforts noted by Kempe & Helfer, 1972).

Retrospectively, it is easy to understand the appeal of such an approach in the early formations of an understanding of child abuse. Because abuse was considered such an unusual and deviant act, it stood to reason that only disturbed individuals would perform such behavior. For many years, there was little understanding of the additional factors involved in the etiology of child abuse, such as the role of difficult child behavior, environmental factors, and the pressures of developing a positive parent–child relationship in the absence of support. Accordingly, the focus was often placed on the parents alone, to the exclusion of important situational events or family members who could have a bearing on the successful outcome.

The underlying assumption guiding such treatment efforts was that abusive parents behaved aggressively toward their children because of their personality disturbance. With the treatment focus aimed primarily at parental (adult) psychopathology, it is not surprising that the early evaluation studies of such treatment were disappointing in terms of preventing further abuse. For example, in the 1970s, the U.S. government evaluated 11 federally funded demonstration programs to determine the effectiveness of traditional methods of lay counseling, parent education, support services, and psychotherapy on the recidivism rates of child abuse. Cohn (1979) reported that 30% of the abusive parents involved in such studies had seriously reabused their children during treatment. Similarly, another study involving 328 families (Herrenkohl, Herrenkohl, Egolf, & Seech, 1979) found that 66.8% of the families involved in their treatment program had incidents of reabuse that were verified. Such failures had occurred despite the fact that one-quarter of the families had received over 3 years of treatment! Thus, it became clear that traditional psychotherapeutic approaches, involving personality change in the parents, were not addressing the problem appropriately (Azar & Wolfe, 1989).

The Influence on Intervention of Large-Scale
Epidemiological Studies

Beginning in the late 1960s, large-scale survey studies expanded
our knowledge of the etiology of child abuse. Gil (1970), working
with nationwide survey data, was among the first to document the
role of poverty and family disadvantage on the rates of child abuse.
These findings were followed by investigations into the social
isolation and chronic stress of abusive families, leading Garbarino
(1977) to propose that isolation from support systems was a necessary, but not a sufficient, condition of child maltreatment. A consensus emerged in which child maltreatment was viewed in relation to economic inequality, because it was reported proportion-
ately more often among economically and socially disadvantaged
families (Pelton, 1978). Furthermore, U.S. statistics were collected nationwide (NCCAN, 1981, 1985) on the sociodemographic characteristics of reported abusive families; as noted in Chapter 1, these revealed that, in comparison to all U.S. children, maltreated children were twice as likely to live in a single-parent,
female-headed household, and four times more likely to be supported by public assistance. Abusive families were also found to
be affected by numerous stress factors, such as health problems,
alcohol abuse, and wife battering (AHA, 1984).

     These illustrative data relating situational factors to rates of
child abuse led to a view of this problem that went beyond the
role of the parents alone. Child abuse began to be defined in relation to its familial and situational context, such as the private and
violent nature of family life and the large number of environmental stressors affecting the family. This viewpoint expanded to
become an "ecological" model of child abuse, which espoused the
importance of the sociocultural context of maltreatment (e.g.,
Belsky, 1980; Garbarino, 1977; Lutzker, 1984). This perspective
argues that as the social structure in which a parent lives becomes
more stressful (or is perceived to be more stressful), the adult may
rely more and more on coercion and violence to control the irritat-
ing daily events that he or she links to such stress.

     One of the most significant theoretical and practical contri-
butions to be made by this emerging sociocultural viewpoint was
that it created pressures to modify the definition and suspected

causes of abuse. Rather than dichotomizing parents as "abusive" and "nonabusive," this perspective was the first to advance the notion that child abuse was more a function of its situational context than it was of an individual's personality weaknesses. That is, child abuse is not an isolated social phenomenon or a personality defect of certain parents per se. Rather, it is a "symptom" of a society that condones the use of some violent methods toward family members, that does not provide adequate services and basic needs for all its members, and that chooses to define maltreatment in relative terms rather than in absolute terms. It follows from this viewpoint that abusive practices are not so much a function of individual disturbance as they are of social and cultural forces that establish the parameters of individual behavior (Wolfe, 1987).

With these new "discoveries" and explanations, some suggestions for improving treatment resources and expanding services to families were offered. Although the ecological viewpoint clarified the causes of child abuse and mobilized some efforts to attack some of its social roots, it was nevertheless difficult to translate some of the causes into treatment or prevention policy. Critics of the status quo definition and policy argued that, because child abuse is a symptom of society, society should attack the elements that create such disadvantages, rather than attempting to patch together the casualties of such societal ills. The implications of this viewpoint for treatment, therefore, may be described in terms of its significance for long-term systemic changes in policy, rather than its influence on current treatment procedures; however, this remains a highly promising and encouraging trend that may have a major bearing on child abuse prevention in the next generation (e.g., Daro, 1990; Wolfe, in press).

The Development of Social–Interactional Perspectives

In the mid-1970s, with the emerging knowledge derived from sociodemographic studies, professionals expressed greater dissatisfaction with definitions that placed major emphasis on parental deviance and wrongdoing (e.g., Garbarino, 1977; Gelles, 1973;

Parke, 1977). This dissatisfaction was due in part to the fact that existing social and legal definitions were aimed primarily at the implicit intent to inflict harm or the incapability of a parent to protect a child from harm. However, research was beginning to suggest that many incidents of physical abuse, although impulsive acts, were not necessarily maliciously perpetrated by the parents. Rather, it was becoming apparent that child abuse was most likely to emerge in those families that lacked the resources and skills to deal with the everyday discipline and stress management issues that constitute a large part of child rearing. Thus, social scientists began to place more and more emphasis upon social and familial variables that could be susceptible to early intervention and treatment.

According to the emerging social–interactional perspective, child abuse began to be viewed as a symptom of an extreme disturbance of child rearing (Burgess, 1979; Starr, 1979), and not necessarily as an individual disorder or psychological disturbance. Abusive families were redefined as ones in which the usual balance between positive and negative interactions and between discipline and emotional bonding has not been achieved. They are families that have ceased to function as facilitators of children's social and cognitive development and that no longer serve as arenas for socialization (Maccoby & Martin, 1983). It was further recognized that child abuse is often enmeshed in other serious family problems (e.g., alcoholism, antisocial behavior), which are all similarly related in some degree to negative developmental outcomes. In light of these definitional and empirical developments, the socialization practices that abusive and other distressed families have in common were pinpointed as areas to receive the majority of attention for defining and treating this problem (e.g., Wolfe, Kaufman, Aragona, & Sandler, 1981).

The social–interactional perspective can to some extent be considered an integration of the concerns expressed by the previous two explanations. That is, this perspective was interested in defining child abuse *in the context of the family, community, and society* (as underscored by the ecological perspective), while also stressing the importance of individual factors that play a role in the actual expression of abusive behavior. Most significantly, the parent–child relationship, rather than individual parental psychopathology or particular stressors, became the target of concern for intervention, because of the belief that this relationship sets the stage for the extent of healthy versus abusive interactions. This perspective not only was influenced by clinical studies of other disturbed populations (e.g., aggressive families; Patterson, Reid, Jones & Conger, 1975), but also benefited from developmental studies relating to the development of parent–child relatoinships, early attachment, and the formation of appropriate child care (e.g., Cicchetti & Rizley, 1981). This view was further influenced by the emerging body of knowledge concerning reciprocal effects of parents and children on each other (Bell & Harper, 1977). The role of child behavior thus became a much more important and significant factor to consider in defining and treating child abuse.

Some of the earlier views of abusive parents as "disturbed" gave way to new empirical findings that embraced a person–situation interaction as the principal factor underlying abusive incidents. In place of personality dimensions, these studies looked specifically at the interactions of family members, as well as self-reports of abusive parents' perceptions of their children, physical and emotional symptomatology that may interfere with parenting abilities, and emotional reactivity to stressful child-rearing situations. Some of the more significant and representative findings from these recent studies are summarized in Table 2.2.

In general, these studies (using comparison groups of physically abusive and nonabusive parents) confirmed the existence of behavioral differences among abusive samples in terms of low frustration tolerance, social isolation, and impaired child-rearing skills. The studies also confirmed several important cognitive differences between abusers and nonabusers, including unrealistic expectations of their children, the tendency to view their own children's behavior as extremely stressful, and their view of themselves as inadequate or incompetent in the parenting role. Interestingly, with the use of matched comparison samples, these studies also revealed that abusive families could *not* be readily distinguished from their nonabusive counterparts in terms of the type and frequency of child behavior problems, the parents' own negative childhood experiences, and the presence of general symptoms of unhappiness or dissatisfaction. Thus, it became

TABLE 2.2. Psychological Characteristics of Abusive Parents Reported in Recent Empirical Studies

---

I. *Behavioral Dimension*
  - Isolation from family and friends (19, 20)
  - Less communication and less child stimulation (7, 8)
  - Disproportionate rate of negative to positive interactions with other family members (3, 4, 11, 13, 16, 17)
  - Failure to match disciplinary methods to child's transgression; intrusive, inconsistent (16, 23)

II. *Cognitive–Emotional Dimension*
  - Self-described as unhappy, rigid, distressed (11, 15)
  - More self-expressed anger (15, 20)
  - Child's behavior perceived as stressful (9, 14, 22, 25)
  - Low frustration tolerance; that is, greater emotional (psychophysiological) reactivity to child provocation (7, 9, 24)
  - Inappropriate expectations of child: disregard for child's needs and abilities; for example, belief that child intentionally annoys parent (1, 2, 12, 20; exceptions: 18, 21)
  - Greater *perceived* life stress (5, 14, 18)
  - Flattened affect during parent–child interactions (16)

III. *Other Findings Related to Psychological Functioning*
  - More physical health problems (5, 11)

IV. *Empirical Findings That Did Not Differ from Controls*
  - Amount of stressful life events (10, 21)
  - Self-expressed emotional needs; for example, feeling unloved; dependency; emotional problems, or personal adjustment (5, 10, 21, 26; exception: 11)
  - Denial of problems (10)

Note. The following studies used matched control groups to compare responses of abusive parents to nonabusive parents from similar backgrounds (see review by Wolfe, 1985): (1) Azar et al. (1984); (2) Bauer & Twentyman (1985); (3) Bousha & Twentyman (1984); (4) Burgess & Conger (1978); (5) Conger et al. (1979); (6) Crittenden & Bonvillian (1984); (7) Disbrow et al. (1977); (8) Dietrich et al. (1980); (9) Frodi & Lamb (1980); (10) Gaines et al. (1978); (11) Lahey et al. (1984); (12) Larrance & Twentyman (1983); (13) Lorber et al. (1984); (14) Mash et al. (1983); (15) Milner & Wimberley (1980); (16) Oldershaw et al. (1986); (17) Reid et al. (1981); (18) Rosenberg & Reppucci (1983); (19) Salzinger et al. (1983); (20) Spinetta (1978); (21) Starr (1982); (22) Susman et al. (1985); (23) Trickett & Kuczynski (1986); (24) Wolfe et al. (1983); (25) Wolfe & Mosk (1983); (26) Wright (1976). The table is from *Child Abuse: Implications for Child Development and Psychopathology* (p. 72) by D. A. Wolfe, 1987, Newbury Park, CA: Sage. Copyright 1987 by Sage Publications. Reprinted by permission of the publisher.

important to view the psychological characteristics of abusive parents in relation to their role as parents and the nature of their families and social contexts (Wolfe, 1987).

Psychological interventions have flourished under the social–interactional model, particularly behavioral strategies (e.g., systematic instruction, modeling, rehearsal, and feedback) designed to assist parents in managing stress in the family context. As summarized elsewhere (Azar & Wolfe, 1989), many of the characteristics of abusive families make behavioral, skills-based learning approaches quite attractive. First of all, the cognitive deficits often found among this population make traditional insight-oriented approaches less appropriate. Behavioral strategies are more concrete and problem-focused, and therefore may be more appropriate for assisting the less intellectually oriented client. In addition, clients' expectations regarding treatment are an important dimension that is matched by behavioral intervention methods. Techniques based on social learning theory are high in face validity and permit clients to work on the problems that are of most urgency and importance to them. Finally, behavioral approaches seem more attractive for this population because parents are often resistant to intervention, at least initially. Because behavioral treatments are often perceived as more "educational" and problem-focused in nature, they may be less threatening to such families and make cooperation a bit easier to achieve.

Over the past decade, intervention methods based on social learning theory and the social–interactional explanation for abusive behavior have focused more and more on developing specific skills for family members, to improve child care and to control impulsive and overly harsh child-rearing methods (for reviews of this work, see Azar & Siegel, 1990; Azar & Wolfe, 1989; Isaacs, 1982; Wolfe, 1987). However, much of this work has focused on children of preschool or early grade school ages, in an attempt to resolve some of the referral concerns that have led most recently to abusive outbursts. Unfortunately, such an application may not be the most beneficial in the long run for this population, because by the time such efforts are begun the parent–child relationship has suffered serious setbacks that go beyond the most observable, presenting problems.

As the following chapters indicate, current efforts are being made to direct the focus of intervention toward the developmental issues that families face during *each* of the emerging developmental stages that the child and parent must endure, rather than attempting to repair the relationship difficulties later on. Such efforts are expanding the focus of intervention to include the early formation of the parent–infant relationship and stimulation of early childhood development, as well as the fundamentals of child-rearing skills.

Summary and Commentary

The preceding synopsis of the theoretical explanations underlying the development of different intervention methods for abusive parents has traced our progress from working with parents individually to working with the parent–child relationship. The field has moved primarily away from a model in which the focus of intervention is placed on the deviance of the parent, and more toward a model in which child abuse is viewed as the result of adult deficiencies *in the parenting role—* in particular, the ability to cope with and manage the stressors associated with this role in a nonviolent fashion. Such a view has led to an expansion of intervention efforts for this population, and more emphasis on early prevention of child abuse through the proper development of parental strengths and resources.

However, it should be noted that most intervention still tends to occur only after a major identified abusive incident, and parents often need a "calling card" of some sort in order to get appropriate help. That is, current laws and priorities are such that child protection agencies have few resources to assist families who have not, as yet, violated any community standard. Unfortunately, our present system is designed primarily for protection rather than assistance, which leaves inadequate services available to the significant number of parents who are at risk of losing control with their children and who could benefit from early intervention. This requires a retooling of our priorities and procedures within the child welfare system, to encourage parents (in a nonthreatening manner) to seek assistance with their role (Wolfe, 1990).

Child abuse is a multifaceted social phenomenon that can be more easily prevented than treated after the fact. This statement follows from the social–interactional definition, which asserts that abuse is a visible sign of serious problems in the parent–child relationship. Such problems typically *develop over time*, and therefore it is crucial to assist families from a point early on in the formation of this relationship, rather than waiting for signs of abuse to occur.

In the following section, some of the effects that abuse may have on children's development are reviewed, for the purpose of highlighting the notion that child abuse is a developmentally linked phenomenon. This developmental link is then applied to a discussion of methods of intervention directed at important developmental "transition points" that may benefit most readily from outside assistance.

The Impact of Physical and Emotional Abuse on Children's Development

In recent years, child abuse research has been enhanced by an expanding knowledge of child development and child-rearing methods. The relationship between early childhood events and child outcome is an important element in developmental psychopathology, and merits the attention it is increasingly receiving in child abuse research (Cicchetti, 1989). Investigators have begun to emphasize that abuse can be defined not only in terms of physical acts to the child, but also in terms of psychological impact on the child's development (Cicchetti & Rizley, 1981; Wolfe, 1987; Zuravin, 1991). Accordingly, physical and nonphysical (emotional) acts of child abuse not only constitute a current parent–child problem, but also may contribute to long-term developmental disabilities for child victims.

Theory stemming from developmental psychopathology suggests that physical and emotional forms of child abuse may interfere with long-term development by virtue of the psychological dimensions that are impaired or disrupted by such parental treatment (i.e., socioemotional, behavioral, and social-cognitive dimensions; see Cicchetti, 1989; Wolfe, 1987). This explanation, moreover, corresponds to findings indicating that physically abused children are more likely to be behaviorally or emotionally impaired than their nonabused counterparts in ways that cannot be attributed to physical injuries alone (e.g., Cicchetti & Rizley, 1981). Such children have been reported to be developmentally delayed, behaviorally disordered, and recognizably different from their age peers, although no particular pattern of psychopathology has emerged (Shaw-Lamphear, 1985). Highlights of these recent findings are summarized below.

Problems Associated with Children's Behavioral, Cognitive, and Emotional Development

Initial studies with children identified as physically abused suggested that such children had higher rates of externalizing disorders (e.g., higher rates of aggression, acting out, hyperactivity, and similar behaviors) than did nonabused children. This finding has generally held up under more rigorous investigation in recent years, leading to the tentative conclusion in recent reviews that physical maltreatment is associated with (but, of course, may not be the direct *cause* of) more aggressive, resistant, and avoidant behavior with adults and peers (e.g., see reviews by Ammerman, in press; Fantuzzo, 1990; Shaw-Lamphear, 1985; Wolfe, 1987). This finding is not surprising, in light of the fact that child abuse comprises physically and emotionally aggressive interactions between caregiver and child, which may form the basis for how the child interacts with others (Sroufe & Fleeson, 1986). At the same time, studies have described abused children as being delayed both in language development (e.g., Appelbaum, 1977) and in their social competence with peers (e.g., George & Main, 1979). Not surprisingly, such children often report greater feelings of hopelessness, depression, and low self-worth (Fantuzzo, 1990).

Despite these overall deficiencies and adjustment problems shown across studies of abused children, there has been little confirmation of the opinion that physical or emotional maltreatment leads to *particular developmental outcomes* for children across their lifespan (Ammerman, in press; Fantuzzo, 1990; Wolfe, 1987). Rather, findings suggest that child abuse represents the visible aspect of a very major disrupting influence in the child's ongoing development. This disruption is so pronounced and significant that behavioral, emotional, and social-cognitive dimensions of the child's development are impaired to varying degrees (Aber & Cicchetti, 1984).

From a developmental perspective, abused children's experiences with their caregivers may have greatest significance in terms of the children's formation of positive relationships with others and contentment in their social environment. For example, the formation of attachment is one of the most critical early developmental tasks; it is believed to set the stage for subsequent relationship formation (Sroufe & Fleeson, 1986). In the field of child maltreatment, the attachment concept has been theoretically linked to the perpetuation of maltreatment across generations (Kaufman & Zigler, 1989), the failure of these children to form subsequent relationships with others (Erickson, Sroufe, & Egeland, 1985), and their vulnerability to failure in additional aspects of development that rely to some extent on early attachment success (Aber & Allen, 1987). Not surprisingly, Cicchetti, Toth, and Bush (1988) report that the vast majority of maltreated infants form insecure attachments with their caregivers (70%–100% across studies). This poor resolution of attachment may be most significant in terms of influencing a child's relationship formation with peers, future partners, and future offspring.

Closely related to the important task of attachment formation is the issue of the development of the autonomous self (at 18–24 months of age). Cicchetti et al. (1988) report that nearly 80% of maltreated toddlers show neutral to negative affect during visual self-recognition experiences. Such toddlers are more aggressive, frustrated, and noncompliant than comparison children in problem-solving tasks that require autonomy. From a developmental perspective, this finding supports the previous arguments detailing the insensitivity of their caregiving environment, and furthermore extends the impact of this insensitivity to the important task of independence.

It has also been determined that abused children show impairments in terms of how they learn to acquire social knowledge. Developmental theorists posit that this is an ongoing process, in which children construct and test social conceptions in relation to personal and social encounters (Shirk, 1988). Again, we find that maltreated children are at significant developmental risk, in part because of the negative and dysfunctional social interactions that they experience on an everyday basis. Because their family members often interact in a physically and verbally coercive fashion, these children have a greater likelihood of learning distorted and maladaptive beliefs about the social world. Such distorted beliefs may further perpetuate their developmental adjustment problems, leading (for example) to an aggressive attributional bias toward peers, or lack of social sensitivity to others (Wolfe & McGee, 1991).

Such findings regarding the broad and diverse developmental disabilities of abused children point to the importance of studying emotional and physical child abuse in terms of socialization practices, rather than individual acts of aggression. For example, physical abuse can be compared to an authoritarian parenting style that is marked by power-assertive, aversive child-rearing strategies (Baumrind, 1971). Consequently, a child's development may be affected most dramatically by the general parenting practices that comprise the child's daily menu of parental behavior. Child abuse, according to this view, may be only the most visible and extreme aspect of an already aversive parent–child relationship. Therefore, the impact of child abuse on a child's development must be considered in relation to the overall quality of care that the child is exposed to over time. Such a view has important implications for early intervention, as discussed throughout this volume.

In a recent review of the literature on the effects of maltreatment on children's development, my colleagues and I (Wolfe, Wekerle, & McGee, in press) have noted two themes among the existing findings. The first theme is that developmental problems among maltreated children appear to be linked most commonly to *poor nurturance* by their caregivers. Thus, it may be more logical to assume that the deficiencies in development among maltreated children are caused by a poor child-rearing environment, of which physical injuries constitute only one aspect. Ample evidence now exists to indicate that maltreated children are poorly cared for, both emotionally and physically, from an early age, and thus it is not surprising to find corresponding problems in attachment and relationship formation.

A second theme to emerge from this literature is that of the *child's response or adaptation to his or her environment over time*. Studies are confirming that children who are maltreated by parents (i.e., physically and emotionally abused or neglected) are more likely than their nonmaltreated counterparts to show signs of failure in normal adaptation. Thus, the way in which such children learn to respond to their environment is closely related to the level of stimulation and sensitivity provided by their caregivers. Because maltreated children are likely to have had poor opportunities to learn appropriate adaptive skills, their reported levels of social competence, self-esteem, and problem-solving abilities are understandably diminished.

In sum, the literature on the impact of physical and emotional abuse on children's development and adjustment reveals that until recently, researchers have approached this issue in a more or less direct, linear fashion. That is, only the physical aspects of abuse were identified, and these were assumed to be directly responsible for developmental outcomes. However, child abuse, like other major situational factors influencing development (e.g., parental divorce, wife assault), may affect development more indirectly through an interaction between the child's developmental abilities and other important mediational factors (most importantly, parental adjustment, family stability, and other compensating or debilitating factors; see Aber & Cicchetti, 1984). Therefore, an important challenge to our understanding of the effects of maltreatment and our concomitant response to this problem lies in our recognition that the effects are dependent on different stages of the child's development and the presence or absence of health-promoting factors (e.g., family stability, alternatives to physical punishment). Such a view necessitates special attention to developmental limitations and abilities of children who have experienced various forms of maltreatment, and provides a strong argument for establishing early prevention and intervention goals.

Implications for Primary and Secondary Prevention

The explanation of how physical and emotional maltreatment affects children has grown from reliance on major and visible signs of trauma to a recognition of the large number of subtle yet crucial ways in which the impact of maltreatment is mediated by the child's course of development. We can now look at some of the implications of these advances in our thinking for primary and secondary prevention of children's mental health problems.

To review, the discussion above has highlighted a prominent theme that links abuse to developmental deviation, which is cumulative over time. Such deviation creates something of a domino effect on subsequent development. From a socialization perspective, "physical abuse" and "emotional abuse" refer globally to the everyday experiences of children that are unhealthy or inappropriate for their physical and psychological growth and development. Frequent or occasional episodes of violence or rejection are not solely responsible for setting in motion children's developmental disparities; rather, this perspective maintains that such episodes are only the most visible markers of a more pervasive concern—a disturbed, dysfunctional parent–child relationship (Wolfe et al., in press).

Such a view can have a significant influence on treatment and prevention directions, in that it takes a somewhat radical departure from most current efforts to treat child victims of maltreatment and to prevent its recurrence. As previously noted, most forms of treatment for child abuse have been directed at parents, once the abuse has been identified. Although treatment of parents and children is a critical and necessary part of service, we need to be aware of the limitations of intervention efforts that take place after abusive patterns of interaction have formed.

If we accept the theoretical and philosophical argument that maltreatment is indirectly responsible for a myriad of developmental problems, then our understanding of the behavioral and emotional adjustment problems shown by maltreated children will rest on such developmental deficits (in addition to some direct effects of maltreatment or insensitive parenting). Such a position carries with it important implications for establishing intervention and prevention goals. First of all, it is important to recognize the developmental differences that may emerge as a function of maltreatment. An individual child's symptoms may be an understandable result of his or her efforts to learn social behaviors without the benefit of sensitive parenting or careful guidance. Accordingly, the identified "referral concern" may shift from one that assesses current problematic behaviors alone toward one that identifies the developmental concerns underlying such behavioral expressions. This premise directs intervention to the strengthening of developmentally relevant tasks or skills, in addition to specific presenting complaints.

Second, we can take advantage of this organizational perspective by seeking to enlist greater cooperation from parents in developing desirable, effective strategies of child rearing, even in the face of competing demands. Instead of relying on aversive contingencies, a developmentally guided intervention and prevention strategy works on the principle of providing the least intrusive, earliest assistance possible. The focus can be shifted away from identifying misdeeds of the parent, and toward promoting an optimal balance between the needs of the child and the abilities of the parent.

Finally, the developmental perspective on the effects of child maltreatment leads to the application of new methods for structuring experiences, in order to help children to succeed in the two prominent areas of development noted previously: the socioemotional basis of relationship formation, and social competence. The objectives of this type of intervention are (1) to strengthen children's self-identity and self-differentiation from an early age, either through improved parent–child relations or through extrafamilial opportunities; (2) to teach social sensitivity and perspective taking in a manner commensurate with the children's level of development; and (3) to provide successful opportunities (for older children) to develop and extend interpersonal skills to relationships outside the immediate family.

An Intervention Model Linked to Critical Transition Periods for Family Members

Despite the numerous suspected and known causes of physical and emotional abuse, these phenomena can be described in terms of a hypothetical course in which abusive and/or neglectful behavior gradually dominates the profile of child rearing. This course largely corresponds to the development of the parent–child relationship, with the exception that such development begins at some point to deviate from the normal or expected course. Child abuse, therefore, can be conceptualized in terms of stages that signify the transition from milder to more harmful interactions over time.

The theoretical viewpoints that have been discussed previously in this chapter offer a number of explanations as to *why* a parent might abuse a child. Although each approach has contributed new knowledge to our understanding of child abuse, further integration of the findings into a transitional model is needed to address the concern of *how* parents gradually acquire the preconditions that seem to lead to the rather sudden onset of abusive behavior. Rather than focusing on observable factors that are often present once a family has been labeled or reported as abusive, this viewpoint looks at the process by which subtle identified contributors to child abuse build up over time to create a situation in which abuse becomes a high risk or an actuality.

The transitional model of abuse (Wolfe, 1987) has been formulated to describe such a course of development in terms that have relevance to prevention and early intervention. The model is based on two presuppositions. First, the development of abusive child-rearing patterns is presumed to follow a more or less predictable course in the absence of intervention or major compensatory factors. This course is described in terms of stages, which serve to underscore the contention that child abuse

DESTABILIZING FACTORS	COMPENSATORY FACTORS

STAGE I:
Reduced Tolerance for Stress and Disinhibition of Aggression

- Weak preparation for parenting
- Low control, feedback, predictability
- Stressful life events

- Supportive spouse
- Socioeconomic stability
- Success at work, school
- Social supports and models

↓

STAGE II:
Poor Management of Acute Crises and Provocation

- Conditioned emotional arousal
- Sources of anger and aggression

- Appraisal of harm/loss; threat

- Improvement in child behavior
- Community programs for parents
- Coping resources

↓

STAGE III:
Habitual Patterns of Arousal and Aggression with Family Members

- Child's habituation to physical punishment
- Parent's reinforcement for using strict control techniques
- Child's increase in problem behavior

- Parental dissatisfaction with physical punishment
- Child responds favorably to non-coercive methods
- Community restraints/services

FIGURE 2.1. A transitional model of child abuse. From *Child Abuse: Implications For Child Development and Psychopathology* (p. 59) by D. A. Wolfe, 1987, Newbury Park, CA: Sage. Copyright 1987 by Sage Publications. Reprinted by permission of the publisher.

develops from a gradual transformation in the parent–child relationship from mild to very harmful interactions. Accordingly, the initial stage is relatively benign in comparison to later stages, in that the parent has not as yet behaved in a manner that significantly interferes with the parent–child relationship. However, this viewpoint suggests that failure to deal effectively with the demands of the parental role at this early point can readily lead to increased pressure on the parent–child relationship and a concomitant increase in the probability of abusive behavior.

The second presupposition of this model relates to the importance of psychological processes that are linked to the expression of anger, arousal, and coping reactions in adults. Specifically, these processes include operant and respondent learning principles for the acquisition or maintenance of behavior; cognitive–attributional processes that influence an individual's perception and reaction to stressful events; and emotional conditioning processes that determine the individual's degree of physiological arousal, perceived discomfort, and self-control under stressful circumstances.

Stage I in this model (see Figure 2.1), labeled "reduced tolerance for stress and disinhibition of aggression," begins with a parent's own preparation for this role (in terms of psychological and social resources, attributional style, modeling, and similar learning experiences from childhood) and his or her current style of coping with daily demands that compete with the parenting role. Parents' responses during Stage I, in which their roles and responsibilities are gradually being acquired, are based largely upon their own families of origin and their preparation for this role through their previous child care experiences. Among those who are at risk of becoming abusive, their training is often inadvertently accomplished over the course of childhood through the modeling of aggressive problem-solving tactics and an external attributional style; rehearsal and reinforcement of aggressive behavior with siblings and peers; and the absence of opportunities to learn prosocial behavior.

Several factors may play a critical role in mediating the expression of aggressive behavior once an individual becomes a parent. In particular, the degree of control, feedback, and predictability that parents perceive in relation to stressful life events can influence their behavior. Stressful events play a critical role in provoking the onset of major health and adjustment-related disorders, and it is reasonable to assume that such events may provoke abusive behavior as well (see LaRose & Wolfe, 1987, for discussion). On a more positive note, however, these difficulties can be counterbalanced by compensatory factors, such as a supportive spouse, socioeconomic stability, success experiences at work or school, and positive social supports upon which the individual can draw for information or assistance (Belsky, 1980; Cicchetti & Rizley, 1981).

Stage II in this model, entitled "poor management of acute crises and provocation," represents the hypothetical point in the development of abusive interactions at which the parent's previous attempts or methods of managing life stress or child behavior begin to fail significantly. The parent often experiences feelings of "losing control," and at this juncture the risk of child abuse (and other forms of poor coping reactions) begins to increase. A parent may "step up" the intensity of power-assertive methods that he or she believes are necessary to re-establish a semblance of control.

Conditioned emotional responding may overtake or impair the parent's rational behavior at this point. Feelings of extreme agitation and irritation, which may have originated from other sources of anger besides the child (e.g., an employer, a neighbor, or a spouse), are (mis)attributed to the child because the parent has learned (through months or years of interaction with the child) to associate feelings of discomfort or irritation with child provocation. (Also, the child is often the easiest party to "blame" for such unpleasant feelings of arousal.) Consequently, when the child cries or fusses to seek attention (for example), the parent may distort the seriousness or potential harm posed by the situation. This appraisal, in turn, may lead him or her to conclude that excessive countermeasures are justified to gain control of the child's aversive behavior. (For a complete discussion of the social-psychological processes underlying this hypothetical set of events, see Averill, 1983; Berkowitz, 1983; Wolfe, 1987.)

Once again, the degree of stress experienced by the parent may be offset by compensatory factors. In particular, improvement in the child's behavior, or the involvement of community programs to assist parents in coping with difficult family-related issues, can go a long way in reducing the acute crisis situation.

The third and final stage in the transitional model of abuse, entitled "habitual patterns of arousal and aggression with family members," represents a chronic pattern of irritability, arousal, and/or avoidance of responsibility on the part of the parent. By this time, the parent may maintain that the use of excessive punishment and force is absolutely necessary to control the child's behavior, or (in the case of neglect in particular) he or she may rely on inappropriate avoidance of responsibility. Provocative stimuli (such as child behavior problems, frustration, and emotional arousal) now become commonplace, and the parent's responses to such events (such as abusive interchanges or neglectful avoidance) escalate in intensity, duration, and frequency.

At this point in time, parents often perceive that they are trapped into continuing to use harsh or extreme methods to control their children. Although this perception is somewhat accurate (because children can habituate to the higher level of punishment and thus may not respond as well to it), the belief justifies their use of further force. Parents are now caught in the vicious cycle of using coercive methods to diminish tension and irritation, and they may receive some short-term gain through such methods by the reduction of the children's aversive behavior.

Unfortunately, the reversal of this process is very difficult at this stage, and is aided by very few compensatory factors (as shown in Figure 2.1). Although treatment efforts may be directed toward families at this point in time, the parents' method of interacting with their children has become so ingrained that it becomes very difficult for them to rely on anything but aversive and coercive methods. One possibility is that parents may become dissatisfied with the use of physical punishment, leading them to seek other ways of resolving child-rearing problems. Furthermore, on occasion some children will respond favorably to noncoercive methods (as a result of either a formal training program or their own increasing maturity), thus reducing the parents' need to rely on aversive contingencies. Finally, community efforts to curtail child abuse may have an impact if a parent is warned of his or her intolerable behavior as soon as a crisis point has been reached, and services are immediately provided to augment the parent's coping resources and reduce the level of stress on the family.

A common dilemma faced by treatment planners is most salient during the third stage. Major efforts to change well-established patterns of family interaction must be introduced in such a manner that a parent will recognize that the benefits (e.g., a well-behaved child or more pleasant family interaction) outweigh the costs (e.g., efforts needed to learn different disciplinary methods, pronounced increases in child problem behavior in the short term).

The task of professionals becomes one of interrupting this deterioration and intervening in such a way as to restore a family's ability to cope with external demands and provide for the developmental and socialization needs of the child or children. According to this view, either the parent–child relationship was never well established from the beginning, or it began to disintegrate during periods of developmental change or family stress. Therefore, an overriding goal of child abuse prevention from the perspective of healthy child development is the establishment of positive socialization practices that are responsive to situational and developmental changes. Such healthy practices serve to buffer a child against other socialization pressures that can be stressful or negative, and reduce the need for the parent to rely on power-assertive methods to control the child.

Methods to assist parents in learning how to be sensitive to their children's development and how to manage their own and their children's behavior more effectively hold considerable promise for child abuse prevention. In the chapters to follow, a comprehensive intervention/prevention strategy that includes such methods is outlined. This strategy has the flexibility to be applied to a greater or lesser extent during any of the three stages in the development of abusive behavior.

3

Selecting Participants
and Introducing Them
to the Program

Presenting Concerns and Responsibilities

In planning an intervention or prevention program for at-risk
families, the obvious fact that the target individuals usually come
to the attention of professionals because of *someone else's* concern,
rather than their own, merits consideration. Due in part to the
nature of child abuse and society's current response to this
problem, it is rare for parents to come forward and indicate their
own need for assistance, especially once they have violated
expected norms or laws. This is an unfortunate state of affairs: Our
laws have created a situation whereby parents are inclined not to
want to identify their problem to others, for fear of losing their
children or somehow being punished or controlled (fears that are,
of course, partially accurate). Therefore, many of the families
coming to the attention of professionals are there as a result of
some degree of coercion (they are usually either court-ordered or
persuaded by child protection agencies).

Most parents who come to the attention of professionals as a
result of suspicions or evidence of child abuse have been reported

to an official agency by someone who has had contact with the families or children. Unfortunately, once again we see that "child abuse" becomes the identified and primary problem, often to the detriment of related and very significant family needs. It is too easy to allow attention to be drawn almost entirely to establishing the validity of the report and the risk of future maltreatment. In principle, the investigator will move beyond the most recent incident of abuse to look at the broader family issues that may be contributing to parent–child problems, although in practice this may not typically be the case (AHA, 1984).

This current state of affairs in North America regarding how parents "enter the system" for assistance in child rearing through reports of abuse requires considerable restructuring if we are to move toward a proactive system that responds to the earlier causes of such violence. Child abuse is viewed throughout this book as a *symptom of family dysfunction*. This view requires that we look beyond the nature of the specific acts of aggression or the individual aggressor, to determine the overall patterns of family functioning. The strategy of assessment presented below is grounded on the principle of family support, rather than identification and labeling of wrongdoing (which in any case is often not the role of the treatment agent). The procedures to establish such support follow from this perspective.

Clarifying Parents' Expectations about a Treatment Referral

There are important issues to address early, both with the referral source and with the parents upon initial referral. Although some parents come to the attention of protective service agencies because of one reported incidence of abuse that is serious enough to warrant a treatment referral, it is more commonly the case that the agency has been monitoring the progress of a family for some time. Such involvement may have arisen from earlier, ongoing concerns expressed by physicians, public health nurses, or others. Evidence of actual abuse or high-risk circumstances may emerge in the context of this monitoring. The parents' belief, therefore, may be that the protection agency is there to threaten them and tell them what to do, rather than to help them. They may complain that their social worker is too busy to talk to them about their particular problems, and that it is only when they lose control and hit their child that they actually receive any "attention" at all.

Although this description is an oversimplification, it does reflect at least part of the reality of what the parents are experiencing. From their perspective, they may see nothing wrong with the way they are handling their child's behavior. In fact, they often draw favorable comparisons to how they were treated as children or how their neighbors treat their children, and therefore feel unfairly targeted by the child welfare system. Most importantly, the parents' defensiveness, although understandable in part, can lead to a digression away from the central problem—conflict in the parent–child relationship.

Because of the nature of the child abuse identification (i.e., "labeling") and referral process, therefore, it is common for parents so identified to be defensive and resistant to efforts aimed at investigating the nature of the problem. When questioned, parents may prefer to relabel the problem as either the fault of their child or a false or unfair accusation. Thus, right from the beginning, obtaining the consent and motivation of a parent/client can be challenging. Several suggestions to improve on this situation are offered below.

Enhancing Rapport and Family Commitment

Initial resistance and defensiveness about allegations of child maltreatment are understandable, especially in light of the fact that acceptable standards of child care are poorly communicated or poorly understood by a significant number of individuals. Some parents have an inaccurate, outdated, and/or limited standard by which to gauge their own behavior toward their children; this often relates to their having been abused or poorly treated during their own childhood. Furthermore, the general acceptance of physical punishment throughout our culture and society supports their belief that what they are doing is neither harmful nor unusual.

To reduce such denial and defensiveness during the initial assessment, an interviewer can focus less upon what the parent has *done* that has led to the involvement of child protective services or other types of actions, and instead focus on what *assistance* can be provided for family members that might help to resolve the current crisis. In other words, an attempt should be made to draw attention toward what a parent may actually choose to address, rather than to attend immediately to the referral or court requirements.

One way to begin this effort is to ask parents to discuss their role with the agency, and to allow them to express openly their feelings or viewpoints about the involvement of other persons up to this point in time. By no means should this effort encourage parents to place blame on others or to allow them a sounding board that could serve to reinforce their views. Rather, the interviewer should permit clients to express their own viewpoint in a *nonjudgmental atmosphere*.

Once the clients have had an opportunity to be heard, the therapist should clarify his or her role with the family, as well as limitations to confidentiality. The therapist should state that he or she can offer some advocacy to family members in terms of their needs, and will make every effort to work with them toward identified goals, *provided the family participates actively*. Because the causes of abusive behavior are very diverse, and because some of the contributing causes for any given family cannot be totally alleviated (e.g., socioeconomic disadvantage, a difficult child), the anticipated goals of intervention must be carefully discussed and agreed upon, to minimize false expectations or overwhelming challenges.

In addition, any responsibility a therapist may have to the referral agent (e.g., the court, protective services, a medical or legal professional) in terms of written reports, discussion of client progress, recommendations for child placement, or the like *must be relayed clearly to the clients* before proceeding further with the therapeutic relationship. Even if a client has "voluntarily agreed" to seek assessment and/or treatment (i.e., without an official court order or other coercion), it is imperative that the limits to confidentiality be stated up front. These limits primarily relate to provisions established by the person's state or province regarding the following:

- The mandatory reporting of *any suspicion* of child maltreatment, defined broadly as a professional's opinion (based on firsthand knowledge or disclosures in the course of treatment) that the child's physical or psychological safety or health (including sexual privacy and safety) is at risk.
- The requirement that the therapist be permitted to share findings with the referral source (as prearranged on an individual basis according to need).
- The possibility of the therapist's having to testify in court about the nature of the assessment or intervention findings, or to discuss the findings at a judicial proceeding (on behalf of either the client, the referral agent, or the opposing side).

In some instances such limits to confidentiality, in conjunction with established therapeutic goals, may best be summarized and made explicit through the use of a written "service agreement" to which the client can refer and review. Such an informal agreement serves the dual role of (1) informing the client about the expected goals of intervention, and (2) clarifying many of the confusing legal and social service agency demands that the client has faced. This agreement should be considered as a confidential document (within the limits stated) and should address pertinent issues between the client and therapist. A sample agreement is provided in Figure 3.1.

Factors Associated with a Smaller Likelihood of Success

At the initial interview and assessment, it is necessary to consider whether or not a family or individual family members are suitable for the type of intervention described throughout this book. Clinical research and experience with the methods described herein have suggested that certain factors make

SERVICE AGREEMENT

Between: _____and _____

Date:_____

In undertaking to assist our family, the therapist agrees to help us explore the effectiveness of our parenting approaches with our son, and to improve in areas that are identified by ourselves and the therapist. In this manner, we hope to assist our child in developing more acceptable and desirable behavior at home.

We agree to attend scheduled appointments regularly (approximately once per week for 2 hours), and to follow through on suggestions provided by the therapist. We will provide the therapist with comments as to the problems and successes we may encounter along the way, to allow for a better "fit" between our style and the therapist's suggestions.

The goals of our involvement, as discussed between ourselves and the therapist, focus on increasing the amount of time we spend with our child, particularly in terms of active play, developmental stimulation, and positive attention. As well, we hope to improve our methods of discipline with our child, in order to reduce our use of criticism, harsh punishment, and anger.

(If applicable or agreed to:)

We agree to permit the therapist to discuss our progress with our caseworker, for the purpose of assisting in case planning and fulfilling our agreement with the agency. A written report at the completion of the program will be provided to our caseworker by the therapist. *We will have the opportunity to discuss in full the contents of this report with the therapist prior to its being sent.*

We understand that any person with whom we may be involved in this program is obligated to report to the child welfare agency any *suspicions of harm or risk* concerning our child that they may have. Such concerns, whether minor or major, will be brought to our attention by the therapist in all cases, in an effort to improve on the situation.

All information from our contacts with this treatment program are treated as confidential, with the exception of information required by law or agreed to by our signature.

Signed, for family: Dated:

Signed, for agency:

FIGURE 3.1. A sample therapist–client "service agreement."

individuals or families less likely to benefit from such intervention.

OLDER-CHILDREN WITH LONG-STANDING FAMILY PROBLEMS

First of all, consideration must be given to the age of the child and the appropriateness of procedures that focus on very fundamental parent–child interactions. In general, the procedures described in this program are most beneficial to parents of younger children, including infants and toddlers. Generally speaking, children over age 6 or 7 will benefit more modestly or more slowly from these procedures. This is not to say that such changes cannot be attempted or achieved, but rather that considerably more effort will be required to achieve relatively smaller gains. This age factor is partly due to the fact that a parent's and child's established patterns of interaction and problem behaviors become more resistant to change over time. In addition, the upper age restriction is partly due to the existence of programs designed more specifically for distressed families with older children. Readers seeking further guidance in this respect are encouraged to review the work of Barkley (1987), Forehand and McMahon (1981), Kazdin (1988), Patterson et al. (1975), and others in relation to conduct problem children and distressed families.

REFUSAL/INTERFERENCE BY EITHER ADULT PARTNER

A second screening consideration relating to the probability of successful outcome is that the adults in some families may view the anticipated benefits of treatment quite differently. One partner may wish to learn about simple games and activities to stimulate child development, while the other is skeptical about people outside the family showing them "how to raise our kids." In dual-parent families, it is clearly more desirable that both partners work together on the program. Alternatively (when either partner refuses or is minimally involved) intervention can involve the motivated partner, as long as the other partner agrees not to interfere or reject the efforts made by the other (and holds to this agreement throughout!). If either parent blocks the other one from actively participating, the referral source must be contacted and informed that the program is not a good match for this family at the present time.

SUBSTANCE ABUSE AND SIGNIFICANT PERSONAL PROBLEMS

Careful screening and monitoring of personal problems that may be principal contributing factors to child abuse are unquestionably critical aspects of assessment and decision making. Although many distressed and disturbed families have such problems to some degree, their existence by no means automatically precludes their participation. The criteria my colleagues and I often use in such cases are as follows: (1) whether the individual responds to our initial interview and observation sessions with some expression of interest, and (2) whether the person shows a minimal ability to care for children. (The initial interview and assessment process are described more fully in Chapter 4.) If problems related to substance abuse, wife assault, or personality disturbance (for example) are of such a magnitude that the individual's day-to-day functioning is very limited or unpredictable, we pre-empt the treatment priorities described herein. In some cases our program can be conducted at the same time as, or following, individualized treatment for these problems. However, one must use extreme caution when implementing the present program with individuals who are in need of a much different type of intervention.

SEVERE AND CHRONIC FORMS OF CHILD ABUSE

Finally, families in which there are very severe or chronic patterns of child abuse, such as incidents involving severe burns or maliciously inflicted injuries, are often not well suited to benefit from structured parent training and methods of enhancing the parent–child relationship. Although this description would seem to apply to the very population of concern, in fact the vast majority of parents who are reported for child abuse have committed acts of a (relatively) minor nature (e.g., harsh or inappropriate discipline, bruises, and related injuries), as opposed to major abuse incidents (e.g., major burns, bone fractures, severe head injuries; AHA, 1984). One study found that in the majority of abuse cases, the reported incident resulted from an attempt to gain control or to "teach" the child (Herrenkohl, Herrenkohl, & Egolf, 1983). Such cases often respond well to structured programs aimed at assistance in child management and anger control (Azar & Wolfe, 1989; Isaacs, 1982). In those remaining chronic and severe cases, it may be necessary to consult with the referral source to consider other avenues of protecting the children (e.g., psychiatric treatment, foster care placement, etc.).

Factors Associated with a Greater Likelihood of Success

Based on outcome studies from our laboratory (e.g., Wolfe & Sandler, 1981; Wolfe, Sandler, & Kaufman, 1981; Wolfe, Edwards, Manion, & Koverola, 1988; Wolfe et al., 1982), as well as studies from related programs (Ambrose, Hazzard, & Haworth, 1980; Azar, 1989; Denicola & Sandler, 1980; Egan, 1983; Hanson, Pallotta, Tishelman, Conaway, & MacMillan, 1989; Lutzker & Rice, 1984; Szykula & Fleischman, 1985) and a study of dropout factors (Wolfe & Manion, 1984), several tentative conclusions can be drawn regarding families who are more likely to succeed in the present intervention program. Successful outcome is generally associated with families in which the following factors apply:

1. A single parent or a couple is experiencing considerable family-related stress (e.g., child-rearing problems) that stems either directly from the child's difficult behavior, or more indirectly from sources of stress impinging on the family. Parents who gain significantly are those who are capable of and willing to focus on child-rearing issues, despite multiple sources of stress in their lives.

2. The parents cannot manage their relatively young child, whom they identify as a source of stress and difficulty. Although resistant at first to being the "focus" of intervention (i.e., because they see the problem as being their child, not themselves),

successful parents are those who generally acknowledge that their current methods have been unsuccessful and who are willing to give something else a try.

3. The parents have a relatively brief record of intervention from or involvement with protective service agencies, either as adults or as children. Often, the carryover from childhood involvement with an agency can involve negative expectancies.

4. The parents show at least some initial willingness to limit their use of corporal punishment and to substitute alternative forms of discipline.

5. Finally, it is helpful, but not necessary, for parents to *identify* (or admit to) the difficulties they are having with their child that stem from their parenting practices, for this will assist in helping them to find alternative ways. The present program does not require that parents label their actions as "abusive" or describe themselves as "child abusers." Because of the often arbitrary and somewhat discriminatory nature of child abuse identification, it is felt that nothing is gained by having parents self-label their behavior with such a global and often misleading designation. In contrast, it is often useful for the interviewer to avoid such labeling and to focus more on the importance of the parents' improving their methods of child rearing, for the benefit of themselves and their child.

In sum, resistance and uncertainty on the part of parents are to be expected in any referral for child abuse treatment. Such reactions should be met by the interviewer with professional acceptance and understanding. From the parents' perspective, they are anticipating that they have been labeled or tagged as some undesirable element of society, and they are often anticipating negative and harsh treatment. Not surprisingly, they are defensive and extremely anxious upon meeting the therapist for the first time. A therapist who greets them with acceptance and a willingness to work with their problems will go a long way in terms of establishing rapport and reducing the resistance that naturally occurs under such circumstances.

Practical Requirements of This Program

Setting and Transportation

The practical requirements for operating this program have been kept to a minimum; they are also fairly flexible, in order to match the resources of different communities, agencies, and individuals. The ideal setting for a family-support-based program such as the one described is one that is familiar and approachable by the majority of clients. This implies that the setting should be located in "neutral" territory that has few, if any, threatening or upsetting connotations (accordingly, space operated by child welfare agencies, criminal justice, or mental health agencies should be avoided in most cases). By necessity, our program has been operating out of a university building (not a counseling center), which unfortunately poses other practical limitations (e.g., distance, parking, and client discomfort and unfamiliarity). Volunteer drivers, who are paid for mileage, provide transportation to many families; this seems to be an essential "first step" in expecting client attendance and effort. An improvement on this arrangement may be to use donated (or leased) space operated by indigenous community centers, churches, or even some schools, as long as client confidentiality is assured. The major considerations affecting choice of location, other than transportation and confidentiality, relate to the availablility of video equipment, observation facilities, and child playrooms, which are described later in the chapter.

Length of Participation

This intervention model has no set number of sessions or hours that must be completed as a criterion for "success." Rather, an intervention continues until such time that the parent and the therapist decide (mutually) that the necessary goals have been reached and problems have been significantly reduced (or, alternatively, the client chooses to withdraw from treatment).

We have found that this is a reasonable structure for most families, because it allows them to "fade out" the program over time, while retaining the option to remain in contact with the therapist over periods of months or years (for assistance in further developmental issues later on).

The exceptions to this open-ended termination policy are the cases in which parents must meet legal requirements. In such instances, we provide the clients and referral source with a clearly stated completion point from the beginning, at which time the achievements of the family will be evaluated and a report can be prepared for the sake of fulfilling a contractual or legal requirement. For example, a family may be required by court to complete a program within 90 days, in order to have the child or children returned full-time to the parents. We establish our goals in accordance with the circumstances, if this is agreeable to all parties. In most cases, judges are willing to return the child(ren) to the family after this time (if the parents are making sincere efforts), and often the family is willing to continue some level of involvement voluntarily, for the purpose of achieving goals set by the program staff.

Selection and Training of Therapists

Most of the therapists (or counselors) for our program have been advanced graduate students in clinical child psychology or developmental psychology. However, we believe that the program's effectiveness does not depend on formal therapist training in these disciplines. On the one hand, given our circumstances, these students have been the most available and affordable, and have considerable knowledge of the training and counseling techniques being used. On the other hand, they lack some of the intangible but significant characteristics that increase therapist credibility and acceptability by the clients (e.g., very few have first-hand child-rearing experience, and their cultural and socioeconomic unfamiliarity to the clients may be initially discomforting to both parties).

Given the realities of personnel cost, training needs, and client characteristics, my colleagues and I maintain that a family-centered intervention program should choose its staff primarily on the basis of interest, motivation to learn and to assist others patiently, and basic familiarity with child care and development. Although staff training is very important, it usually cannot substitute for a person's basic comfort with and understanding of small children. Teaching parents ways to interact with their children more favorably often requires a flexible, trial-and-error approach that depends to a considerable degree on the experience and skill of the therapist. This viewpoint is compatible with the use of senior citizen volunteers, child welfare agency staff or volunteers, or indigenous paraprofessionals (we have no firsthand experience in training these groups, however).

Staff training begins with new therapists' being paired with experienced therapists, and observing the procedures with different families over time. Simultaneously, they are assigned readings in child development and parent training (e.g., Forehand & McMahon, 1981; Maccoby & Martin, 1983; Patterson, 1982; Sroufe & Fleeson, 1986) and in child abuse intervention models and procedures (e.g., Azar & Wolfe, 1989; Wolfe & Manion, 1984; Wolfe, Kaufman, et al., 1981). Before the preparation of the present volume, therapists were provided with written guidelines for conducting weekly sessions. I have altered this week-by-week therapy structure herein to focus more attention on the major objectives in each phase, and to reduce the overreliance on weekly assignments or tasks.

We no longer formally attempt to train our therapists in specific child management techniques (e.g., time out, removal of privileges, reinforcing incompatible behavior), but rather prefer that they choose from the wide range available (through reading and experience) in an effort to match their own preferences most closely to those of their clients. We have found that the nature of teaching positive methods of child discipline and sensitivity to parents is highly personalized in many instances, and thus it is important to avoid becoming too reliant on specific methods. Therapists are exposed to many different forms of child discipline and teaching strategies during their training, and are observed applying their preferred methods with parents. Ongoing supervision of therapy sessions is conducted: Either live or videotaped excerpts then are reviewed by more experienced professional staff.

Introducing Families to the Clinic

The first assessment and first therapy sessions are undoubtedly the most critical and stressful for all family members. Because of this fact, and the likelihood that families will drop out or resist involvement unless they feel that they "fit in the program," we strive to introduce the program, staff, and setting in a manner that is sensitive to their initial apprehension and ambivalence.

Parents and children are given a full tour of the facility on their first arrival at our clinic. They are brought into the playroom, which contains a cupboard full of toys and an open area for joint play or talking. One-way mirrors and hanging microphones are immediately obvious upon entering the room, and so we explain their purposes by taking them behind the one-way mirror and showing the equipment that we use. Parents and children are assured that no one else will be viewing them from behind the one-way mirror without their knowledge and permission, and the purpose of the equipment and room arrangement is explained (i.e., to allow one party to observe the others less obstrusively). Younger children, below age 4 or so, usually take little note of the equipment or the mirror. Older children, on the other hand, are quite fascinated by it and may want to spend some time investigating its function.

Most importantly, we show parents and children how the video equipment works, because it is an integral part of the intervention program. We inform them that we like to videotape sessions some of the time, and we explain (and provide a written assurance) that these tapes will be available only to themselves and to the treatment staff. Tapes are kept locked up, and no one is permitted to use or view them except members of the project staff. (This agreement covers social workers and other individuals not on the project staff, who are not informed of the existence of the tapes. However, parents are again reminded that we are obligated to comply with legal requirements for reporting suspected abuse, and to provide subpoenaed materials.) With their consent, such videotaping affords a record of progress the family is making over time. I discuss the additional clinical benefits of this taping in sections to follow.

Parents are informed that sessions generally run from 1 to 1½ hours, and that they are free to take a break at any time. We establish a simple rule that any toys removed from the cabinets have to be replaced before the family leaves. Because this setting is designed primarily for younger children (the playroom is 5 meters by 5 meters, with a small observation and video room adjoining), parents seem to find things to do with their children quite easily. We avoid the use of interview rooms that might make them feel ill at ease, and prefer instead to let children choose the initial activities to break the ice. Moreover, once parents see the video equipment and have an opportunity to watch themselves on tape, the vast majority are comfortable in allowing this procedure.

Because it is common for children to act out during the initial meetings, we prefer to have parents and children remain together in the playroom and simply play together until both become more accustomed to the setting (with the therapist joining in gradually). As part of the intervention strategy, we prefer to postpone any efforts aimed at controlling or modifying a child's behavior until such time as the parents have become fully engaged in the program (i.e., the parents are beginning to attend to the child and to improve their positive expressions and actions toward the child). Needless to say, however, children may seize this opportunity of greater parental attention and lessened control to misbehave during these early sessions, leaving parents in a situation in which they feel immediate help is needed. In addition, parents will often bring to the session problems that have been occurring at home during the past week, and expect immediate guidance. While supporting their desire to bring forth these problems, the therapist tells the parents that a foundation for change must be created before any substantial improvements in child behavior can be expected. They are reminded that "kids' behavior often gets worse before it improves," and that this is a sign that the intervention is on the right track; that is, their child is responding to changes in parental attention and the like, and this marks the start of learning more desirable behavior.

These issues notwithstanding, staff members must be prepared to offer assistance in the home immediately (often with the help of someone from the social agency, such as a homemaker or parent support worker) if the parents feel that this is necessary for them to cope with existing problems. If a situation does emerge at home that merits some immediate assistance, the order in which components of the program are presented can be modified at the discretion of the therapist to assist parents in managing the crisis. Although my colleagues and I caution that this is not the preferred method (because it creates a greater chance of overall failure, in that parents may not learn the prerequisite skills to solving new crises), occasionally this is a clinical decision that is made in order to keep a family from dropping out of treatment, or to avoid the eruption of major conflict in the home.

Establishing Peer Group Support and Social Services

Old habits of overreacting to children's curiosity and activity levels die hard. Because of this fact, it is critically important that a parent and child be given every opportunity to establish more pleasant, enjoyable patterns in their relationship. In addition to the provision of such opportunities, the success of treatment can often hinge on being able to hold the old patterns and major disrupting influences (e.g., frequent changes in housing, employ- ment, or partners; high levels of daily stressors) in check long enough for new ones to take hold. This is where support services, provided in conjunction with the present training program, play a crucial role.

Families who are involved in our treatment program also participate in group activities twice each week. These activities are operated by the local children's protective services, but they are provided in a neutral location by child care specialists (not protective service social workers). The meetings are organized to encourage friendship and social support, rather than formal counseling or therapy. Although groups are predominantly attended by single mothers (due to the fact that our community has focused on this needy population), male partners attend on occasion.

These informal activity groups are also attended on occasion by former "graduates" of the training program, who provide additional reassurance for parents that things can improve with effort. A member of our program staff attends these groups periodically to address particular group concerns (e.g., dealing with former partners, handling temper tantrums, etc.) and to observe how parents assist one another. We further rely on this support group to provide parents with additional feedback or encouragement in their efforts.

The group meetings also allow children to have an opportunity to play with peers and to strengthen some of their developmental skills. A day nursery is housed in the building, and is staffed by two child care workers who are trained to teach children's prosocial behaviors. Thus, the nursery permits parents to bring their children to group meetings—and, more importantly, to observe their children interacting with peers, to speak to child care workers about their children's development, and to discuss their children with one another.

As further community support for the training program, we ensure that parents are offered assistance by the community on an "as-needed" basis. Parents are able to bring their children to a respite center for a few hours or overnight. This permits them to take a break from any tension at home, or simply functions as a support service to permit single parents, for example, the opportunity to choose responsible alternatives for babysitting and personal pursuits. We believe that this respite program provides an important "safety net" throughout the treatment program. The center is operated independently of protective services, and families can use the service on their own initiative. Most importantly, the staff members at the respite center are trained to observe both children and parents, and to share their observations in a constructive way with families and program therapists (on consent).

Thus, throughout the treatment program, parents are involved in three forms of intervention. First of all, they meet on a weekly or regular basis with a therapist and receive individual guidance and direction for establishing a more positive relationship with their children. Second, they meet on a regular basis with peers; this provides an opportunity to spend time with other adults, to strengthen their social supports, and to receive feedback and encouragement for learning new child rearing behaviors. Finally, they are offered a respite center in the community that is aimed at providing a safety valve for families who may lack the resources to take needed breaks from their children on a regular basis. This center is staffed by persons who are familiar with the training project, and therefore reinforce the parents' attempts to follow through with the efforts being made.

4

Identifying Parental Expectations and Treatment Priorities

The formulation of any intervention strategy always requires a careful assessment plan; this is particularly true when one is dealing with high-risk families. Because each family has very different needs and resources, it is important to conduct a broad-based assessment. Typically, this involves obtaining information from multiple sources, conducting careful interviews with the parents and perhaps the children, and observing family interactions. This chapter explores some of the ways in which these things can be done, with emphasis on those issues of assessment that require particular sensitivity on the part of the assessor.

Because child abuse potential can only be partially assessed through questionnaires or tests, this chapter does not focus on any particular psychometric devices. Rather, it presents a strategy for assessment that relies primarily upon clinical skill, careful interviewing style, and thorough knowledge of the issues related to this problem. This is not to say that certain tests or questionnaires may not be advantageous at times. Those individuals who are trained to administer personality measurement devices may find them helpful in understanding the contribution of an adult's personality in the expression of abusive behavior. However, there are few norms available for abusive parents upon which to draw conclusions, and therefore caution must be exercised in interpreting such test findings.

A notable exception to the above-noted lack of psychometric devices for high-risk populations is the Child Abuse Potential Inventory (CAPI; Milner, 1986). This instrument was developed specifically for use with abusive and at-risk adults, and its psychometric properties have been documented with this population. The CAPI provides useful screening information for exploring an individual's background, his or her particular attitudes about child rearing, and any attempts on his or her part to distort responses in an attempt to appear well adjusted. The major strength of the CAPI lies in its ability to identify potential areas of weakness or risk that require intervention, as well as its utility in highlighting particular background factors that warrant closer assessment. However, the test developer cautions against relying primarily on this or any other psychometric instrument for the purpose of detection or confirmation of child abuse; additional information is essential for such investigations. Interested readers should consult recent reviews of psychometric tests with abusive populations for further details of the advantages and disadvantages of such devices (e.g., Milner, 1991; Wolfe, 1988).

I now turn to some ways of assessing general problem areas among these families; this is followed by discussion of parents' child-rearing methods and a focus on children's needs.

Assessing General Problem Areas

Assessment Purposes

Child abuse treatment referrals are usually made to assist in pending decisions by child protective services concerning child placement and parental "rehabilitation," and/or decisions by the court concerning the possibility of a less intrusive disposition than severance of parental rights. Some of these pending decisions can benefit greatly from the information provided by the treatment agent, especially if he or she carefully weighs the alternatives for the family and child, and points out to both the family and the referral agent any reasonable expectations that may follow from treatment involvement.

Determining dangerousness and risk to children in cases of detected or undetected maltreatment is one of the most common purposes for assessing abusive or high-risk families. Such an assessment is used to assist in determining whether or not to take a child from a family or to place the child in an alternative setting. Because the assessor brings to the situation background knowledge of and experience in understanding factors that are critical to healthy child development, it may be his or her role to balance a proposal to remove a child with knowledge relating to the risk such placements may pose to the child's well-being and to the family's long-term stability.

Removing the child from the family for the sake of protection carries with it the formidable risk of breaking apart the (fragile) parent–child relationship. Once separated, the parent, the child, or both parties may be incapable of addressing the problems in the family; they may seek only to be reunited (for further discussion of this crucial issue, the reader is referred to Garbarino, 1987; Jones, 1987; Melton, 1990). Thus, an assessment can be very useful to determine whether the parent, the child, or both are capable of dealing with the crisis that has arisen from a child abuse report without resorting to further violence.

A second important assessment purpose is to identify the general strengths and problem areas of the family system. In most assessment situations it is important to identify what major factors preceded the abuse, and which factors may maintain such abusive behavior in the family if left unabated. This information provides direction for protective services, support, or additional community services. However, the advantages of involving different service providers must be carefully weighed against the potentially overwhelming demands on the family. In addition, the different crises that family members report may change dramatically, requiring a considerable shift in the direction of intervention.

The interview should proceed from a discussion of general family background and particular family problem areas, toward a discussion of parents' individual difficulties in managing child-and family-related issues. Such an assessment often requires several different sessions before the interviewer is completely familiar with the family situation.

Because of the multifaceted nature of child abuse and high-risk child-rearing circumstances, assessing such families requires attention to a broad number of issues. The following subsections identify different general problem areas and provide suggestions as to how to gather such diverse information. It is important to emphasize that each of these areas is necessary in assessing high-risk families, because each represents potential elements of risk that may need to be thoroughly understood and perhaps addressed in subsequent intervention. An outline summary of these issues is presented in Table 4.1.

Individual and Family Background

A discussion of each adult's background is an essential foundation for intervention planning; yet this can raise resistance and discomfort for many parents under the present circumstances. Surprisingly, most parents are willing to discuss memories of their own childhood, once they recognize that the interviewer is not attempting to place blame for the present situation, but is sincerely interested in hearing about such experiences. Often their memories include harsh or severe treatment by their own parents or surrogate caregivers. Although parents are less likely to identify themselves as having been "abused" per se, quite often they describe childhood experiences that make their own inappropriate behavior pale by comparison.

This aspect of the initial interviewing process is essential in building rapport and understanding the current family context. Moreover, in some circumstances such discussion may actually be therapeutic for some parents, because they have actively avoided discussing their own childhood trauma or memories. Such avoidance, and the accompanying distortion of significant traumatic events, often result in chronic, diffuse symptoms of distress and discontent (i.e., negative affectivity; Watson & Pennebaker, 1989). An opportunity to discuss their childhood

TABLE 4.1. Parent Interview and Assessment Guide: Abuse and Neglect

The following is a selected summary of the major factors associated with child abuse and neglect, requiring further interviewing and assessment of the parent, as indicated. The framing and emphasis of each question are left up to the discretion of the interviewer.

I. Identifying general problem areas
   A. Family background
      1. Early rejection or abuse during own childhood; relationship with biological and/or psychological parents
      2. Methods of punishment and reward received during own childhood
      3. Family planning and effect of children on the marital relationship
      4. Preparedness for and sense of competence in child rearing
      5. Early physical, emotional, behavioral problems of child (i.e., illness, trauma, temperment)
   B. Marital relationship
      1. Length, stability, and quality of present relationship
      2. Examples of conflict or physical violence
      3. Support from partner in family responsibilities
      4. Substance abuse
   C. Areas of perceived stress and supports
      1. Employment history and satisfaction
      2. Family income and expenses, chronic economic problems
      3. Stability of occupation, income, and living arrangements
      4. Perceived support from within or outside of the family
      5. Daily/weekly contacts with others (e.g., neighbors, social workers)
      6. Quality of social contacts and major life events (i.e., positive vs. negative influence on the parent)
   D. Symptomatology
      1. Recent or chronic health problems; treatment; drug and alcohol use
      2. Identifiable mood and affect changes; anxiety; social dysfunction
      3. Previous psychiatric evaluations or treatment
II. Assessing parental responses to child-rearing demands
   A. Emotional reactivity
      1. Perception of how particular child differs from siblings or other children known to the parent
      2. Feelings of anger and "loss of control" when interacting with child (describe circumstances, how the parent felt, how the parent reacted)
      3. Typical ways of coping with arousal during/following stressful episodes

(continued)

TABLE 4.1 (continued)

B. Child-rearing methods
  1. Parental expectations of child (i.e., accuracy of expectations for child behavior and development, in reference to child's actual developmental status
  2. Examples of recent efforts to teach new or desirable behavior to child
  3. "Preferred" and "typical" manner of controlling/disciplining child
  4. Attitudes toward learning "different" or unfamiliar child-rearing methods
  5. Perceived effectiveness of parent's teaching and discipline approach
  6. Pattern of child behavior in response to typical discipline methods (i.e., accelerating, decelerating, manipulative, responsive

Note. From "Child Abuse and Neglect" (p. 652) by D. A. Wolfe, 1988, in E.J. Mash and L.G. Terdal (Eds.), *Behavioral Assessment of Childhood Disorders* (2nd ed., p. 652). New York: Guilford Press. Copyright 1988 by The Guilford Press. Reprinted by permission.

associations with someone who listens with interest and concern can turn into the beginning of a positive and beneficial therapeutic relationship.

The particular issues that should be addressed in such an individual interview include a discussion of any early rejection or mistreatment during childhood, as well as the adult's retrospective view of the relationship with his or her biological and/or psychological parents. Such information appears to be very predictive of parents' current coping styles and personal adjustment (e.g., Main, Kaplan, & Cassidy, 1985), and serves to establish the parameters of how they deal with problems with their own children. This discussion can include methods of punishment and reward, as well as any particularly memorable childhood experiences (both positive and negative). How parents describe and rate their own childhoods, therefore, often reveals important issues bearing on their current child-rearing perspective.

Recent and current family matters can be best covered through a joint interview with both parents in a two-parent family, either preceding or immediately following the individual interviews. Of most significance to this interview is the couple's description and appraisal of family planning efforts and the effect children have had on their marital relationship, lifestyle, and expectations. Their preparedness for family life and their sense of competence in the child-rearing role can then be reviewed.

As noted previously, the CAPI (Milner, 1986) may be useful during this initial stage of the assessment to help identify concerns or issues from the parents' own childhoods. Similarly, the Parenting Stress Index (Abidin, 1983) helps parents to describe all of the current sources of stress in their lives, either related directly to a child's behavior or related more to events affecting the parents and the family in general. It is natural for parents to express both doubt and frustration in adjusting to their changing role; raising these struggles can be useful in determining the parents' willingness to consider alternative ways of handling such stress.

Finally, both parents' knowledge of and interest in a child's early physical, emotional, and behavioral problems should be reviewed at this point. In particular, any illnesses or physical trauma a child may have experienced, and their views of the child's early temperament, are important topics for discussion in formulating an understanding of the early parent–child relationship.

Marital Relationship or Partnership

Following discussion of the family background, it is useful to see each partner individually to discuss his or her views of the marital relationship or partnership. This usually begins with a discussion of the length, stability, and quality of the present relationship as each partner perceives it. It is particularly important to identify any examples of unusual conflict or physical violence in the relationship, because if either partner feels threatened or harmed by the other, his or her responses to other aspects of the assessment will be compromised.

Wife assault is believed to occur in approximately 40% of cases of physical child abuse in which both partners are living in the home (Jaffe, Wolfe, & Wilson, 1990; Straus, Gelles, &

Steinmetz, 1980). Thus, it may be necessary to address marital violence prior to addressing violence toward children. This assessment can be formalized by using measurement devices such as the Conflict Tactics Scales (Straus et al., 1980), or can be completed simply through questioning both partners concerning how they "typically" resolve conflicts, and how often they may engage in physical or verbal fights over issues (e.g., the frequency of yelling, hitting with objects, throwing things, etc.).

The interview with adult partners should also address the extent of perceived support each receives from the other partner in terms of family responsibilities. It is often the case that only one partner (usually the mother) is involved in the vast majority of the child-rearing responsibilities—a state of affairs that can lead to greater stress in the family and a higher likelihood of abuse among predisposed families. Finally, during individual interviews, it is important to assess the possibility of any substance abuse by either partner. A history of alcohol or drug use should be taken, and a determination should be made as to whether or not such problems preclude the involvement of the family in parent training programs.

Areas of Perceived Stress and Support

How family members perceive their current situation, both within the family and within the community at large, has a great bearing on how comfortable they are in the child-rearing role. Furthermore, major stressors on a family, such as unemployment or loss of income, are known to provoke incidences of child maltreatment. Accordingly, parents may be interviewed concerning current sources of stress, both to identify their significance and to determine how the family copes with them (whether they occur on a daily basis or unpredictably). Potential areas of stress include, for example, employment history and job satisfaction; family income and expenses, as well as chronic economic problems; and a discussion of the stability of the wage earner's occupation, income, and living arrangements. It is not uncommon to find that the family has moved a number of times in recent months, which also contributes to tension and disorganization within the family.

Along with such discussion of perceived stress, parents may be asked about sources of support they perceive from within or outside of their family. Such discussion usually centers around whom they speak to on a regular basis, whom they confide in, and whom they visit frequently for social purposes. We often ask about the quality of their social contacts, to see whether or not they enjoy such contacts or whether they find them to be stressful (e.g., some parents say that they do not enjoy visiting other relatives and would rather be left alone). The identification of very few perceived sources of support raises questions as to the parents' ability to form and utilize informal or formal support networks, and indicates the need to address this issue early in treatment.

Psychological Adjustment and Symptomatology

The final general problem area to be assessed is that of any major physical or psychological symptoms reported by either parent, or observed by others. Again, this is best done during an individual interview with each parent, in which he or she is asked about recent or chronic health problems and their treatment, as well as distressing emotional or behavioral symptoms. Any mood or affect changes, anxiety symptoms, or social dysfunctions need to be identified through interview procedures, followed up by psychological testing. A psychiatric history of evaluations or treatments, if any, should also be obtained on consent of the client. Although the presence of such symptoms (including a formal diagnosis of psychiatric illness) does not necessarily preclude an individual from benefiting from the present treatment program, it is essential that such problems be carefully weighed prior to initiating an intervention strategy that focuses on improving the parent–child relationship.

The results of our work with this population concur with the general finding that severe psychopathology (e.g., schizophrenia, major depression, sociopathic personality) is relatively rare among samples of abusive parents (5%–10%; e.g., Kempe & Helfer, 1972; Wolfe, 1985). However, such parents quite often report a number of physical and psychological *symptoms* that, although not of sufficient severity to constitute a "disorder," can clearly interfere with progress in treatment unless recognized and managed. In the present program, we emphasize the importance and benefit of parents' strengthening their child-rearing abilities even in the presence of elevated symptomatology, as long as such symptoms are being managed medically or psychologically as well as possible. Quite often, parents reduce their levels of distress as they learn to enjoy and become more effective in their parenting role.

Assessing Parental Responses to Child-Rearing Demands

I now turn to parents' specific responses to the child-rearing role. Particular areas of concern include their emotional reactivity and their child-rearing methods. Both of these concerns can be addressed in the first instance through careful interviewing, and then can be further assessed during observations of parents' interactions with their child.

Emotional Reactivity: The Assessment of Anger and Arousal

Because child abuse, by its very nature, involves uncontrollable emotional reactions and rage, a careful assessment must be conducted of the manner in which a parent manages emotional arousal and anger. This sensitive topic can be approached by asking parents to describe how a particular child differs from siblings or other children known to the parent. Parents who hold a distorted view of their child will often describe him or her in extremely negative, unrealistic, and overly harsh terms (Azar, Robinson, Hekimian, & Twentyman, 1984). Such negative attributions are usually associated with anger, and can often lead to rage if a parent has no way of managing such feelings.

At a more specific level, we ask parents to describe in detail feelings of anger and loss of control they have experienced during exchanges with their children. To facilitate this self-monitoring task, we ask them to describe recent circumstances in which they have felt annoyed or frustrated, and to describe exactly what they thought and felt and how they reacted to the children.

Most parents have no difficulty describing such situations; In fact, we find this to be an exercise that enhances their involvement with and commitment to the intervention program. Parents seem to appreciate being able to tell the therapist about problems that their children "cause" them, and ways in which a particular child upsets them. Such a discussion leads naturally to clarifying their typical ways of coping with arousal during and following such stressful episodes. In this regard, the interviewer focuses on the manner in which parents determine that they are aroused or stressed by a child, such as elevated heart rate, "seeing red," shouting uncontrollably, or similar signs of losing control. Generally speaking, parents who are able to identify the first stages of losing control in some fashion are well on their way to benefiting from subsequent intervention.

Parents may also be asked to keep an "anger diary" for 2 or 3 weeks at home. Such a diary simply asks them to record situations during the day in which they become angry at a child, and to denote what event(s) preceded the situation and what they did about it. Parents may also wish to identify how they felt throughout the situation, and to record how pleased or disappointed they were regarding their reaction (see Wolfe, Kaufman, et al., 1981). Self-monitoring is a crucial aspect of intervention, and a diary facilitates parental involvement in such monitoring. Needless to say, however, some individuals will not readily accept this self-monitoring "exercise," and thus the examiner must rely more heavily on the interview and information obtained from parents' retrospective descriptions of recent crises involving children who angered or provoked them.

The assessment of anger, in many circumstances, is distinct from the assessment of aggressive actions toward a family member. Whereas some individuals may be willing and able to discuss identified feelings of anger, others may resort to aggressive tactics with little or no self-described buildup of arousal and tension. In addition, a person may easily "displace" his or her anger and arousal onto another source (usually a convenient family member, such as a spouse or a child), without recognizing the original source(s) of irritation and anger (Averill, 1983; Berkowitz, 1990). For example, a father may return home after a bitter argument with a coworker, and the arousal from this previous confrontation can be transferred to his interaction with his child. At the slightest provocation, the father may overreact to the child and potentially become abusive. Such displacement or transfer of arousal, moreover, can occur over time to such an extent that the original source of anger is several steps removed from present circumstances (e.g., anger at one's own parents).

For these reasons, we have found that the assessment of anger and aggression should be conducted simultaneously, in a fashion that allows for an identification both of (1) the person's perceived source of the anger (whether accurate or misattributed), and (2) his or her *preferred* and *actual* ways of coping with the anger. To assist this task beyond the interview stage, my colleagues and I conduct ongoing observations of each parent's expression of verbal and physical aggression as part of each subsequent contact, based on our general understanding of the person's anger profile that was determined from the interview.

Because this treatment program involves parent–child contact throughout, such observations are conducted as part of the regular sessions with the family. An observer chooses a somewhat demanding task in which to engage a parent and child, and then notes how the parent expresses frustration and irritation and how he or she copes with such arousal. The parent is encouraged to talk openly during such an observation (in which the observer is located behind a one-way mirror and unknown to the child), ostensibly to "inform" the observer of the difficulty he or she is having with the child, but also to re-enact situations that occur at home that may lead to anger and aggression. Over the course of an intervention, this observation becomes more routine, and consequently more revealing of the parent's degree of interfering emotional reactivity to child behavior.

Those individuals who recognize the inappropriateness of their reaction, and in fact report unpleasant distress and discomfort when angered, are distinctly the best candidates for intervention. In our experience, these individuals account for the majority (75–85%) of adults involved in our program. *Ipso facto*, those who deny such feelings, or who attribute their feelings and actions entirely to external forces and not to themselves, are likely to resist any effort expended toward identifying and managing their sources of anger and arousal. These latter individuals may require another therapeutic direction, one that places greater emphasis on the identification and appropriate expression of anger (see, e.g., the discussions by Berkowitz, 1990, and Brewin, 1989), preferably followed by a program in child-rearing methods similar to the one described.

Child-Rearing Attitudes and Methods

Assessing the specific methods that parents use to control or teach their children usually begins with a discussion of a parent's expectations of a child. The interviewer should note whether these expectations are accurate in terms of the child's actual behavior and developmental status. We also ask about recent examples of efforts to teach new or desirable behavior to the child, and the child's response to such efforts. Parents are also interviewed about their "preferred" and "typical" manner of controlling and disciplining children. Quite often, parents indicate that they have used "every method available" in an attempt to control their children, so it may be useful to discuss how they handle situations in which the child requires some structure and discipline, on a day-to-day or hour-by-hour basis.

Parents are also asked about their attitudes toward learning "different" or unfamiliar child-rearing methods. Most parents are resistant at first to discussing their child-rearing style, because they construe such discussion as leading to criticism and fault finding. However, they are more willing to do so if such discussion is presented in a manner that focuses on areas of desired change or improvement *in a child's behavior*.

This discussion of child-rearing attitudes and preferences can be bolstered by asking parents how effective they believe their teaching has been with their children, as well as how effective their discipline has been. According to a recent Canadian survey, most parents (even those who adhere to corporal punishment) admit that such methods work only occasionally, and that they become overly angry and upset each time they punish (Institute for the Prevention of Child Abuse, 1989). Moreover, many parents can detect that their use of physical or overly harsh forms of discipline has gradually increased over a span of time, requiring them to use harsher methods each time in order to produce the same result. Thus, some disillusionment with physical punishment may be uncovered if such discussion is couched in a nonthreatening, nonjudgmental manner aimed at looking for alternatives.

Finally, it is useful during the interview to discuss how a child usually responds to the parents' typical discipline methods. Once again, parents often prefer such discussion, in that this gives them an opportunity to point out to the interviewer how difficult their child can be and how much assistance their child "needs."

Clinic and Home Observations

To facilitate assessment of parents' emotional reactivity and child-rearing methods, parents and children should be observed together while engaged in different activities. We conduct such observations in our clinic, because we can provide the necessary "props" and can limit distraction. This observational task begins by asking a parent to play quietly with a child and to make every effort to attend to whatever activity or interest the child prefers (if both parents are present, usually one parent at a time sits in with the child, while the other observes). We are interested at this point in viewing how comfortable and capable the parent is during an activity with the child in which the parent is *not in control*, but rather is merely attempting to show interest in the child's play. Although this is a low-stress situation in principle, some parents appear to be uncomfortable in this passive role, and reveal their need to show more control and authority with their children.

After several minutes of this low-stress interaction, we ask the parent to teach the child a new game or activity appropriate to the child's developmental level. Parents usually enjoy this shift toward greater structure and control, which allows them to display their ability to maintain direction of their children. Of course, we are most interested in the methods they use to instruct, guide, encourage, prompt, reward, and perhaps punish or control the children throughout this teaching task. We take particular note of the "emotional tone" of these interactions (e.g., the degree of parental enthusiasm, voice clarity, harshness, irritation, etc).

Lastly, we ask the parent to have the child put away the desirable toys, and to play only with one remaining (and less desirable) toy for a few minutes. Not surprisingly, this request often sets into motion a more stressful interaction, marked typically by child noncompliance and emotional out-bursts. This contrived situation thereby permits observation of how each parent handles such common predicaments, as well as a firsthand view of how difficult the child can become if he or she is redirected away from a desired activity. Once again, it is expected that the situation will be quite difficult for both a parent and a child; however, we see this as an important opportunity for parents to reveal to the treatment staff just how "difficult" their children can be. That is, this moderately stressful situation permits parents to receive some much-needed confirmation for their claim that *their children* are very difficult and require treatment. During this initial assessment stage, it is important simply to acknowledge such a need, while emphasizing that in order for children to improve their behavior it will be necessary for parents to try other forms of discipline and encouragement.

At the conclusion of each and every clinic visit, the parent and child are given an opportunity to play quietly again and restore their composure. If for any reason parents appear to remain angry or perplexed, we confirm with them that either a member of our staff or their social worker will visit them shortly to follow up on the visit and see how things are going. If this is communicated in a concerned fashion that avoids any sense of blame or failure, parents may appreciate, rather than refuse, such follow-up contact.

At the same time, it is also advisable to visit the parent and child in the home several times during the assessment period to permit a better understanding of the family situation and to determine firsthand how chaotic or confusing the home life may be to the child. During home observations we usually initiate only low-stress situations of play or teaching games, because the higher-stress situations will usually emerge on their own (e.g., bedtime, finishing a meal, getting dressed, etc.). Not only does the home observation provide an excellent opportunity to view the child's behavior and the parent's reaction to such behavior in the natural setting, but we find that it also helps to establish better rapport with the family.

Both qualitative and quantitative data are collected during these observations in the home or clinic. This data collection is aimed at determining the frequency and quality of parenting methods that favor the child's social and cognitive development, as well as identifying the functional relationships between parent and child behavior. Observers should choose a recording method that assesses the major dimensions of parenting that are conducive to intervention. These dimensions include verbal and physical positive behaviors, criticisms, commands, and verbal and physical negative behaviors, as well as the "affective delivery" of these behaviors (e.g., voice tone, orienting the child to the task, age-appropriate language and directions, interest in the child's response, etc.). At a minimum, observers or therapists should record the interactions descriptively by writing a condensed narrative of the interchanges. More formally, they can record their observations on a criterion-based checklist that lists many of the desirable child-rearing behaviors to be observed and taught (e.g., the Parent–Child Interaction Form; Wolfe, Kaufman, et al., 1981), or a structured observation form that permits ongoing recording of chosen behavior categories, such as commands, criticisms, and so forth (see Wolfe & Bourdeau, 1987, for review and discussion of these various approaches). For most clinical purposes, a careful recording of the interchanges, in reference to appropriate and inappropriate parenting behaviors, is sufficient to determine goals for treatment.

Assessment of the Child

Abused and neglected children require specific assessment, in addition to the observations of them during interactions with their parents. For the most part, the assessment is directed toward an understanding of the child's developmental disabilities, problem behaviors, and other impairments that are related to a history of maltreatment. Therefore, the assessment must be tailored to the individual developmental level of each child.

The discussion to follow covers child assessment under two major headings: (1) the child's behavior with other family members, and (2) the child's adaptive abilities and cognitive and emotional development. It is assumed that the assessor may choose to add standardized tests to evaluate the child's adjustment and development in other areas (such as intelligence, physical and motor development, etc.).

Child Behavior with Family Members

How children interact with other members of their families is a critical aspect of assessment prior to intervention with abusive families. By and large, a child's behavior in the family is a function of the extent of coercion and aversive interactions that have been going on for some time; therefore, assessment of child behavior involves observations of the child during interactions with family members, as well as parental report.

Parents' reports on their perceptions of a child's behavior are particularly useful, even though they may not be accurate descriptions of the child's actual behavior. Obtaining these reports is a relatively straightfoward procedure: Parents are asked to indicate problem areas that they have been experiencing with their child, and in particular to note how they want such behaviors to change. Often it is useful to administer a global child behavior inventory, such as the Child Behavior Checklist (Achenbach & Edelbrock, 1983), to provide a backdrop for some of this discussion. Because the purpose of this assessment is to determine the extent of the parents' distortions of the child's behavior, as well as to obtain a standard of comparison for the child's behavior with other family members, parental reports are weighed against situational factors that might bias such reports or distort such findings (e.g., degree of contact with child, desire to make child "look disturbed," etc.).

A child's behavior during interactions with family members can be assessed in much the same format described above in relation to parental emotional reactivity and child-rearing methods. However, to obtain a more thorough observation of the child's strengths and weaknesses, the situation may be additionally structured to involve a task or activity that is somewhat difficult for the child to complete, in an attempt to see how the child handles such a task (as well as to see how the parent handles this task). For children under age 6, we conduct a structured parent–child observation in our clinic as well as at home. This observation proceeds in much the same way as described previously: We begin with a low-frustration, minimal-contact activity in which the parent simply follows the child's activity and interest. This task then begins to shift after 10 or 15 minutes to involve more parental direction and compliance tasks.

A useful variant on this technique is to add a distraction task for the parent, especially for children under age 4. The parent is asked to complete a checklist or to engage in some other activity while the child is playing with a low-interest toy on the floor. Because the parent is distracted in much the same way that he or she would be at home when on the telephone or cooking, the child may seize this opportunity to be more demanding and attention-seeking. We find that such opportunities to observe children under realistic circumstances are well received by parents, because they are glad to have others witness the difficult situation that they must deal with at home.

For older children who have reasonable verbal skills and listening abilities, this observational situation can be modified to involve a structured parent–child discussion of a problem issue. The parent and the child each identify an issue, such as completing homework (parent issue) or reducing yelling (child issue), and they are given 15 minutes to discuss each issue and possible alternative solutions. This procedure, which has been used successfully with parent–adolescent conflicts (Foster & Robin, 1988) provides ample opportunity to observe the problem-solving skills of both the adult and the child, as well as to witness the emotional tone that each party displays during conflict resolution.

Children's Adaptive Abilities and Cognitive and Emotional Development

Even very young abused children often lag behind somewhat in their development, as a function of the inadequate child-rearing stimulation that they have received. Thus, for younger children of preschool age, we often conduct a standardized assessment of their intellectual and social development in an attempt to determine the degree of developmental deficiency or lag. Such an assessment involves standardized testing and observation of a child while he or she is engaged in tasks related to physical and sensory development. Interested readers may consult Sattler (1988) in reference to conducting such assessments with younger children who may have experienced negative life circumstances.

Once children are old enough to be interviewed and to provide information about themselves, a wealth of important data can be gathered. A semistructured interview with a child is a particularly useful method for beginning to elicit the child's feelings, beliefs, and attitudes pertaining to family, self, and school. For a child from an at-risk family, the interview should lead to a discussion of the child's perception of discipline, changes in the family, and other current events. The following objectives may be kept in mind when conducting such interviews:

1. Children's own perceptions of recent family events and crises that have occurred are assessed. Children often have opinions of their own regarding what has happened, and this leads to the formation of an attributional process that may be maladaptive later on (e.g., "This happened to me because I'm a bad kid").

2. Children's perception of blame or responsibility for the crisis or recent events are evaluated. In addition, children may be asked to discuss their families' future and what changes they would like to see in their families.

3. Children's perceptions of each individual family member are discussed, in terms of each person's roles in the family, use of appropriate or inappropriate discipline, and the setting of rules. Children are often quite protective of their parents during such discussion, and may provide information that contradicts the social work investigation. The reasons for this are poorly understood, but it should be recognized that young children (under age 8 or so) often blame themselves for parental anger (e.g., Covell & Abramovitch, 1987). Thus, children may reframe an abusive situation in terms that put the blame on themselves. Children above age 8 or so may be more likely to comprehend situational cues in discussing the use of inappropriate discipline and parental anger in the home, and so the interviewer can seek to discover what cues a child may identify to explain parental behavior (e.g., parental drinking, parental arguments, etc.).

4. Safety skills with children, which include their comprehension of unsafe situations and actions they would take to protect themselves in such situations, are reviewed. Safety skills such as those that would be involved in a fire, a fight outside of their home, and a fight that involves family members are of foremost importance.

5. Children are interviewed regarding their attitudes toward violence and conflict. School-age children, in particular, may have quite distorted views about violence (both in the home and outside of the home); we also get a diversity of responses from males and females concerning the appropriateness of violence, the extreme fear of violence, and similar widely discrepant reactions. We ask children to apply this perception of violence to peer situations if appropriate, in order to determine the extent to which they have begun to use such attitudes to deal with peer-related conflict.

6. Children's levels of social skill and social competence are assessed by observing their verbal abilities and problem-solving abilities throughout the observation and interview. We are particularly interested in determining whether children have alternatives from which to choose in the event of frustrating or conflict-laden situations. Those children who are capable of seeing different, nonviolent solutions are at a lower risk for future peer conflict and conduct problems in most cases.

The administration of self-report instruments and structured diagnostic interviews with children can serve a related purpose of identifying adjustment problems, developmental differences, and emotional reactions among this population. The choice of such instruments is quite broad, and must be narrowed down according to particular concerns noted by the interviewer (see Hansen & MacMillan, 1990, and Wolfe, 1988, for suggestions of particular psychometric devices).

Because of the unique experiences of this child population relative to other child clinical populations, it is valuable to use a structured interview technique aimed particularly at children's post-traumatic-stress-related symptomatology and coping reactions. A colleague and I (Wolfe & McGee, 1990) recently developed such a tool for evaluating children's (ages 8 and older) perceptions of events in the family, and the presence or absence of major symptomatology related to these events.

We are finding that children who have undergone a lengthy history of emotional, physical, and/or sexual maltreatment by their caregivers often have developed beliefs and coping styles quite different from those of average children, and that these coping styles merit careful attention. In particular, some children have learned to suppress emotional symptoms, a process that seems to create considerable discomfort as well as maladaptive coping responses (Pennebaker, 1985). For example, symptoms related to post-traumatic stress—such as intrusive memories of particular events; heightened arousal and fear when children are reminded of such events; avoidance of activities, places, or people that remind them of particular events; and physiological symptoms that impede their day-to-day activity—may be of such magnitude that they warrant individual treatment.

Children (usually 4 years and older) may be asked about symptoms of intrusive thoughts, escape and avoidance reactions, and physiological reactivity during a structured interview in relation to traumatic memories and/or identified traumatic events. At the same time, children are asked how they usually cope in the presence of such symptoms, and how successful their methods of coping have been in easing the symptoms. For example, children may report that they have nightmares in which they see a figure chasing and attacking them. Commonly, children report that they cope with such repeated nightmares by "trying to forget them," which in most cases results in the problem's growing worse over time. Similar coping reactions are often seen in many other stress-related situations; therefore, one aspect of treatment for children may involve relaxation training, counterconditioning of phobic or fearful reactions, or group or individual counseling to deal with such symptomatology (see Wolfe, Sas, & Wekerle, 1990, for examples of this concept with sexually victimized children).

In sum, the present overview offers general guidelines for assessing child victims of maltreatment, although methods will vary considerably according to the individual needs of each child. Both visible signs of developmental disparities (such as behavioral adjustment problems) and less visible signs of emotional turmoil (such as post-traumatic-stress-related reactions and emotional symptomatology) may be present in children who have been maltreated. Assessment of such children, therefore, involves an ongoing process aimed at identifying the presence of some of these adjustment disorders.

Linking Assessment Findings to Treatment Considerations

Some of the following points are summarized from the discussion throughout this and previous chapters, in an effort to link assessment findings to treatment planning; others expand upon points previously made.

A major difficulty in any intervention with an abusive or high-risk family is the establishment of parental compliance and motivation for treatment. Initial roadblocks can be reduced by coordinating the goals of treatment carefully with court and/or agency goals as described in the referral. This coordination should take place prior to any involvement of the family in a treatment program, to ensure that all parties agree upon and have a clear understanding of expectations. In some cases, it is useful to prepare a written "service agreement" stipulating objectives, time frame, and consequences (positive as well as negative) that have been arranged among the therapist, the client(s) and the referral source.

As a further suggestion for minimizing initial resistance, referral problems can be reframed in terms of day-to-day difficulties that a parent is having with a child, to avoid the often unnecessary implications of labeling the parent "abusive." Parents may be more willing to work at changing day-to-day problems with their children because this is a concrete and identifiable concern, whereas they are often confused about and unwilling to address problems that *others* have identified. Preferably, parents will seek further individual counseling at a later date to address some of the underlying factors contributing to child maltreatment, although we must realize that such counseling may be alien to the thinking of and ill suited to the needs of this population (Aronson & Overall, 1966).

Abused children have special needs that require unique assessment and intervention planning. Because these children have been attempting to adapt to difficult situations, changes in family arrangements or process should be made gradually and carefully. One suggestion is to establish a working relationship with each child prior to introducing any changes in child-rearing style. This can be done through gradual play activities or other low-key interactions, until such time as the child is able to become involved in activities with the parents.

Furthermore, aggressive and problematic behavior that the child may display should be approached in a calm and matter-of-fact manner, despite the fact that this will not always be immediately effective. Children from abusive families may act out considerably, once they are in a setting that is unfamiliar or appears to be more "safe." These periods of acting out should be seen as opportunities for the therapist to demonstrate for the parent how to respond to difficult situations without becoming explosive or abusive. Finally, a "cooling-off" period must be introduced after any stressful procedures have been conducted with the parent and the child. Family members should be allowed to engage in a mutually enjoyable activity, such as playing games or watching themselves on video playback, to permit them to regain composure and overcome any anger that may have been provoked.

Therapists must also deal with stressful demands placed upon the therapeutic relationship, because working with abusive and at-risk parents creates considerable "role strain" and "agenda conflict" (Azar & Wolfe, 1989). To deal with such demands, professionals working with this population need to be able to manage their own personal reactions to parents' past behavior with their children. It is essential for assessors and therapists to attend to parental actions and attitudes in a nonjudgmental fashion, while at the same time avoiding the appearance of condoning such behavior. In addition, an assessor or therapist must cooperate fully with protective services and gain a working relationship with the agency, in order to follow through on some of the suggestions that emerge from assessment. Limits to confidentiality should be carefully explained, and mutual consent should be obtained among the referral source, the family, the child (if appropriate for his or her age), and the therapist prior to beginning any assessment or treatment procedure.

Once the period of assessment is coming to a close, it is time to establish reasonable goals and expectations for change with the family as well as the referral source. At this point, many treatment decisions that relate to the client, the format of treatment, and any support personnel who may be available must be made. The therapist may wish to emphasize more of a parent focus as opposed to a child focus, or alternatively may find that working with the child first is more crucial because of the child's developmental or motivational problems. Although the program described in the chapters to follow is designed primarily for individual families, therapists may consider different formats such as group or dyadic treatment (involving one parent and child, or both marital partners), in conjunction with clients' particular interests and needs.

By and large, the program described herein is one in which goals are chosen for an individual family, and both parents (or one parent, in a single-family home) work together with the child. Group meetings (usually operated by the local child welfare agency on a weekly or biweekly basis) are highly desirable for the purpose of developing social support and additional skills at problem solving. Although group meetings are not usually the best arena for attempting actual behavior change with at-risk parents, they may serve a valuable role in establishing common concerns and social support for this population.

Finally, the therapist must establish priorities among the diverse family needs that inevitably arise in conducting an assessment. The treatment program described herein is quite flexible in terms of when and how it can be administered; yet such an approach would not be the first priority in cases in which there is significant alcohol or drug abuse, ongoing wife assault, criminal behavior, or other activities that may lessen the relative importance of child management training. Although the referral agent has often identified such problems and perhaps screened out certain families prior to referral, it is the therapist's ultimate decision as to whether or not a family can benefit at present from this program.

5

Intervention: I. Methods for
Promoting Parental Sensitivity
and Responsiveness
to Child Behavior

(with ANNE KRUPKA)

The treatment programs described herein are founded on the belief that promoting a *positive and responsive parent–child relationship* is both a desirable intervention target and a viable child abuse prevention strategy. Accordingly, the procedures used to achieve this goal range from highly structured interactions with the child (involving specific stimulation techniques and child management techniques) to more loosely structured opportunities for parents to rehearse their own style of interacting with the child in a more positive fashion. In addition, because child abuse is marked by impulsive, stress-related reactions to the child, our program involves an anger control component that is tailored to the needs of each parent individually. Most importantly, these methods are intended to be used to assist families in a flexible manner that is sensitive to cultural differences and realistic limitations of change.

Currently, the view that child maltreatment is a "relational failure" resulting from a dysfunction in the parent–child–environment transactional system is gaining wide acceptance (Cicchetti et al., 1988). Such failure is thought to be due to the presence of debilitating factors (poverty, adolescent parenthood, single parenthood, etc.) that place extra burdens on the parent–child relationship, as well as to the absence of proper social support and guidance. Accordingly, increasing numbers of researchers and practitioners are focusing on the quality of early interactions between children and parents who are at high risk for child abuse and neglect, with *prevention* of maltreatment as their goal.

The rationale for such programs is straightforward: Many at-risk families with very young children (under 24 months of age) are not yet experiencing the serious child behavior management problems that bring their counterparts with preschool-age and school-age children to the attention of child protection agencies. Parent–child interactions are still relatively benign, although subtle indications of future problems may be present. If parents can be reached at this early stage, the chances of influencing patterns of parenting and promoting healthier parent–child relationships are improved, and the likelihood of future child abuse and neglect is diminished.

For a variety of reasons, young, socially disadvantaged parents often lack the skills necessary for effective parenting. Many lack knowledge about infant development and therefore have inappropriate expectations for their infants' behavior in the first 2 years of life. They tend to overestimate the rate of development and often become impatient and intolerant when their infants fail to live up to these expectations (see Miller, 1988, for a review). When interacting with their infants, they usually display relatively low levels of affect. When they do engage in affective interactions, they tend to display more inappropriate and negative affect (Hann, Osofsky, & Carter, 1990).

For adolescent or immature parents in particular, their own stage of development (e.g., poorly defined personal identities, self-centeredness, the inability to anticipate the needs of Sothers) can increase their risk of maltreating their children.

Thus, programs that help young parents to enjoy their parental role serve simultaneously to promote feelings of self-worth and effectiveness, which in turn enhance behavioral sensitivity (Lamb & Easterbrooks, 1981). If such parents' relationship with their children is happier, the increased sense of enjoyment can make the parents more receptive to basic child-rearing information.

To attain the necessary and important goal of child abuse prevention, new programs and new ways of presenting them are needed. Most existing clinic-based intervention programs for child-related problems place a strong emphasis on parental control and management of the target child. However, such an emphasis may be less appropriate for parents who themselves have been identified as the principal concern, or for parents with children under 2 years of age. The topics and examples used in most parent training programs (discipline and control issues) may not be as developmentally relevant for younger children, or may not fit the needs of multi-stressed, immature parents.

This chapter describes our approach to teaching parents to be more sensitive to child development and behavior. Following a discussion of the role of parental sensitivity in effective parenting, we first present procedures that are especially designed for parents of toddlers and infants, followed by the objectives and methods pertaining to parents of preschool-age children. In general, these procedures form a flexible, nonthreatening, child-centered treatment program to help parents and children achieve mutually enjoyable interactions, which allows parents to "start over" and learn some of the most basic and fundamental ways of teaching and enjoying their children.

The Role of Parental Sensitivity in Effective Parenting

Prominent theories of development assign a major role to parental sensitivity in the social, emotional, and cognitive development of the child. As noted by Lamb and Easterbrooks (1981), parental sensitivity is "perhaps the most important determinant" of individual differences in infant social cognition (p. 127). At the very least, parental sensitivity is basic to the provision of adequate care and a stimulating psychological environment for infants (Wiesenfeld & Malatesta, 1983). Although parental sensitivity can be operationally defined in different ways, there is general agreement that the concept involves the ability of a parent to provide *contingent, consistent, and appropriate responses to the child's or infant's signals*. Parents exhibit sensitive behavior when they perceive their infants' cues, interpret these cues correctly, and respond in an appropriate and effective manner. In contrast, insensitive parental behavior results when there is a deficiency at any point in this process (Lamb & Easterbrooks, 1981).

Parental sensitivity facilitates optimal child development in many ways. Parents who exhibit high levels of sensitive behavior provide their children with information and intellectual stimulation through verbal interactions. They allow their infants physical freedom to explore the environment without undue restriction or control, thereby encouraging the development of sensory and motor abilities. They support their infants' and toddlers' budding sense of self by responding to their needs in a manner that is consistent with their developmental level. Furthermore, they strengthen the children's self-esteem through positive affect, which accompanies all their supportive verbal and physical interactions (Wolfe, 1987). Despite its recognized importance, however, relatively little is known about the antecedents of parental sensitivity. Maternal responsivity and receptivity to infants have been shown to vary with maternal perception of stress (Loyd & Abidin, 1985), as well as with infant's prematurity (Frodi & Lamb, 1980), developmental level (Brooks-Gunn & Lewis, 1984), delayed language development (Wurlbert, Inglis, & Kriegsmann (1975), and handicapping condition (Fraiberg, 1974; Wedell-Monnig & Lumley, 1980).

Just as there is empirical evidence linking maternal sensitivity to optimal infant outcomes, there is also empirical evidence linking maternal *insensitivity* to child maltreatment (Crittenden, 1988; Egeland & Sroufe, 1981), to insecure attachment (Ainsworth, Blehar, Waters, & Wall, 1978; Smith & Pederson, 1988), and to lowered levels of cognitive development (e.g., Bornstein & Tamis-LeMonda, 1989; Coates & Lewis, 1984;

Lewis & Coates, 1980). Atypical infant behavior patterns have been associated with maltreatment as well, although it is difficult to determine whether these behaviors are the cause or result of abuse.

Methods for Enhancing Parental Sensitivity:
A. Infants and Toddlers

Training parents to be more sensitive and responsive to their infants' signals and needs is a relatively recent endeavor. Although the techniques to date are derived primarily from applications with nonabusive parents, and from programs with all female and no male participants, the following discussion illustrates some of the innovative ways that therapists can assist parents in learning how to interact with their small children in a positive and mutually enjoyable manner. Expanded or modified versions of many of these techniques form the basis for the intervention goals described for preschoolers in the next section.

Infant-Centered Activity and Stimulation Techniques

Mahrer, Levinson, and Fine (1976) describe a technique they call "Watch, Wait, and Wonder" for promoting infant-centered activities with mothers. (Unfortunately, information on father participation in this and many other stimulation programs is lacking.) The baby is placed on the floor of a therapy room containing toys and is allowed to explore. The mother is instructed to get down on the floor with the baby and watch what he or she does. The mothers is further asked not to initiate activity or interfere with the baby's exploration, and is instructed only to "watch, wait, and wonder." Persistent initiation by the mother or a lapse into a traditional caretaking mode ends the session. Each interaction is videotaped, and the mother is asked to critically evaluate what has taken place. A major benefit of the program, as reported by staff members, is that the mother's relationship with her baby becomes a happier one, and she becomes more aware of her own style and significance to the infant.

Long-Term Home-Based Intervention Methods

Olds and Henderson (1989) have pioneered a comprehensive home-based intervention program for reducing the rate of maltreatment among high-risk families. Trained nurses visit mothers approximately once every 2 weeks during the last trimester of pregnancy, and then on a varied schedule until the infants are 2 years of age. They prepare mothers for labor, delivery, and early care of their newborns, and they teach parents the importance of a healthy pregnancy and responsive caregiving for optimal physical, cognitive, and socioemotional development in children. Rather than focusing specifically on maternal sensitivity and the attachment relationship, the nurses try to improve the mothers' understanding of their babies' need for responsive caretaking. In addition, they seek to enhance the mothers' informal support by encouraging husbands, boyfriends, and other family members to participate in the home visits and by assisting parents who want to go back to school, find work, use effective birth control, or find appropriate community services. Their initial findings, based on first-time parents who were teenaged, single, and/or low-income, have been quite supportive of this home-based, ongoing service for preventing maltreatment and parent–child relationship problems.

Short-Term Center-Based Interventions

Short-term, goal-specific programs also show merit in assisting the formation of a positive parent–child relationship. Crittenden & Snell (1983), in 4 months of weekly intervention sessions in a group setting, taught disadvantaged, at-risk mothers to use the "facing position" when socially interacting with their infants. Mothers were instructed to take their infants to a small blanket spread on the floor and to play with them. Toys and an infant seat were available nearby, but no further instructions were given about how the dyads were to behave. Intervention consisted of replaying 1-minute videotapes (previously recorded of each mother–infant dyad) for the entire group to observe and discuss. Each mother's position relative to her baby, and its effect on her own and her baby's behavior, constituted the focus of the group discussion. Modeling and role playing, in addition to the discussions, were used to help mothers learn to change their position during intervention. Improvement in a mother's position relative to her baby was related to increases in both maternal interactional behavior and infant development.

Short-Term Home-Based Intervention

An abuse prevention project for young, socially disadvantaged mothers and their 3-month-old babies is currently being evaluated by Krupka and Moran (1991). Like the programs noted above, this project is aimed at improving early mother–infant interactions by enhancing the mother's sensitivity to the signals and needs of her child. The training has several purposes: (1) to reinforce the strengths already present in a mother's behavior; (2) to increase the mother's awareness of how her behavior influences her baby's behavior; (3) to increase the mother's awareness of her baby's cues and needs; and (4) to establish positive experiences for both the mother and the baby. The ultimate goal is to increase the mother's sensitivity to her baby so that she reads his or her cues accurately and responds in a contingent and appropriate manner, thus facilitating the establishment of a secure infant–mother attachment relationship.

An 8-level hierarchy of parental interactional behaviors, ranging from least to most sensitive behavior (based on the work of Clark & Seifer, 1983), provides both the framework for examining maternal behavior and the guidance for teaching mothers to interact with their babies in increasingly adaptive and mutually satisfying ways. Play interactions videotaped in two assessment visits 1 week apart are rated on 5-point scales (ranging from high to low) for each of the eight categories. The ratings, based on the frequency and intensity of the behaviors in question, determine the levels at which a mother routinely interacts with her baby. During 40-minute, biweekly sessions, the therapist helps the mother move up the hierarchy of interaction behaviors (described below). Mothers are taught the appropriate behaviors that they do not use consistently through videotape feedback, verbal instructions, modeling, and use of positive reinforcement. Intervention sessions continue until a mother routinely interacts with her baby at the highest level in the hierarchy of sensitive behaviors.

Strategies for intervention focus on mother–infant play interactions, and follow as closely as possible those suggested by Clark and Seifer (1983). At the beginning of each intervention session, a mother and her baby are videotaped for 1 minute. The mother is asked to play with the infant on a small blanket spread on the floor. Toys are available for the mother's use, but no further instructions are given about how the mother and infant are to play. The mothers is told:

> Play with your baby in any way that you like. We are interested in observing the way mothers and babies play with each other. We have brought a few toys that you may use if you wish. Just do what feels comfortable.

The tape is then viewed by the mother and therapist, and the mother is reinforced for those behaviors that are conducive to good interaction (e.g., eye contact, voice changes, etc.). Attention is then focused on behaviors that need to be modified. The therapist requests permission to try some changes that might improve the mother–infant interaction. (Clark and Seifer have found this step to be very important in establishing rapport.) The therapist discusses and models the appropriate behaviors, and the mother is then encouraged to try interacting with her baby in the specified ways for another 1-minute videotaped interaction. The mother is told:

> Don't worry if you forget some of the suggestions. Most mothers do. We will coach you when necessary. For example, if your baby needs to be reinforced for vocalizing and you happen to forget, we will ask you to acknowledge or imitate the vocalization.

While viewing the second 1-minute videotape, the mother is encouraged to talk about the things that she notices during the interaction, and she is again given feedback regarding her own behavior and its effect on her baby's behavior. The mother is asked to play with her baby in the suggested manner for approximately 3 to 5 minutes three times a day during the 2 weeks between sessions. Mothers are given cards with illustrations and descriptions of the exercises to be practiced, and on which they can record the duration of each play interaction.

The intervention procedures used by Clark and Seifer (1983) to help mothers of handicapped children move up the hierarchy have been modified by Krupka and Moran (1991) for use with young at-risk mothers. Because this hierarchy is germane to the specific intervention techniques, a description of the eight levels is provided:

1. *Uninvolved*. Intervention with mothers who demonstrate minimal eye contact and/or minimal smiling begins by having the mothers carry their infants and note signs of hunger, discomfort, or contentment. Mothers are encouraged to recognize differences in infant crying behavior, so that they will not misinterpret the babies' cries either as signs of caregiving failure or as indications that the infants are intentionally trying to annoy them. Close physical contact in the early months of life not only makes a mother more aware of her infant's needs and states (Anisfeld, Casper, Nozyce, & Cunningham, 1990); it enhances her ability to interpret cues correctly and to respond more appropriately.

A mother's position relative to her baby, and its effect on her own and her baby's behavior, ares also emphasized at this level. Mothers who look at their babies "en face" normally provide more infant-initiated stimulation and more reponses to infant-initiated behavior than mothers who sit beside or behind their babies (Crittenden & Snell, 1983). Mothers who do not interact in a face-to-face position do not have direct access to eye contact. Such a mother is taught (a) to face the baby so that each has easy access to eye contact; (b) to make eye contact and smile when the baby looks at the mother; (c) to make eye contact and vocalize when the baby looks at the mother and vocalizes; and (d) to notice when the baby averts his or her gaze, and to stop smiling or vocalizing then.

2. *Forcing*. This behavior occurs most frequently in mothers

who are anxious about their babies' development or who are insensitive to their babies' cues. Such mothers may engage in excessive touching, talking, and head movements. When a baby begins to fuss and turn away, a mother may hold the baby's face in midline to re-establish eye contact and begin a new interaction. (Clark & Seifer found that showing videotapes of such interactions without the sound was helpful, as mothers were able to focus more easily on their babies' signals when not distracted by dialogue.)

Some very young mothers treat their babies as dolls to play with, rather than as separate beings in need of nurturing. They pick up their babies whenever they feel like playing with them, and put them down when they themselves grow tired of play. They tickle, jiggle, and prod to get their babies to perform some action of their choosing. They know that babies must be fed, changed, and put to sleep, and usually do a good job of tending to the infants' physical needs. However, the agenda they follow is their own, not that of the babies'. To get these mothers more "in tune" with their babies' agenda, the "Watch, Wait, and Wonder" technique described above is used. The mothers are also introduced to imitation as a means of following their babies' lead. The important aspect here is teaching a mother to become a good observer of her baby's behavior. Mothers begin by imitating each vocalization and each facial expression (e.g., yawn, smile, open mouth, frown, eyes wide, etc.). If they feel self-conscious imitating some behaviors (e.g., hands or fingers in mouth, arms flailing), mothers can choose not to imitate them. (Clark & Seifer found that mothers became more relaxed once they were assured that the slowed-down, exaggerated quality is the important aspect of imitation.)

3. *Overriding.* Mothers interacting at this level appear to have difficulty monitoring their babies' signals, a skill necessary for sensitive caretaking. These mothers may spontaneously interrupt the infants' ongoing behavior or try to direct the babies' attention to a new activity. They often have difficulty in allowing breaks in the interaction. At this level, conventional infant games are used to teach a mother to become more aware of the ways in which her particular baby is signaling his or her needs. The mother is taught to wait for the baby to look at her before beginning the game, to pause when the baby looks away, and to wait until the baby looks

at her to continue the game. In this way, mothers learn to observe the wide range of responses their babies exhibit, and to slow down and wait for their babies' response. (Clark & Seifer found "Tell Me a Story" to be particularly effective with overriding mothers. In this game a mother asks a child to "tell a story," and then uses any facial expression, gesture, body movement, or vocalization as a piece of information for the story. She responds with comments such as "Oh, really," "You don't say," "Imagine that," and "What else do you have to say?" Any baby response is sufficient to keep the game going.)

4. *Involved.* Mothers at this level attempt to engage in mutual eye contact and mutual smiling. They take pleasure in what their babies are doing, but may have difficulty engaging the babies. A variety of intervention strategies are used for mothers at this level, depending upon the deficits in the mothers' repertoire of interaction behaviors. Some mothers may need to be taught the importance of maintaining eye contact (by asking them to respond only to eye contact and to ignore all other behaviors for a short period of time). Others may need to learn how to read subtle cues of waning attention and fatigue (by reviewing videotapes for yawning, glassy eyes, fidgeting, fussing, etc.), or how to use specific infant attention-getting behaviors and chain behaviors to sustain interest (by reviewing videotapes for wide-eyed expressions; looks of anticipation; smiling, shaking, or nodding of the head; rhythmical, repetitive gestures or vocalizations; etc.). Mothers who show little or no game playing are taught typical infant games ("Itsy Bitsy Spider," "I'm Gonna Get You," "Pat-a-Cake," etc.).

In addition, taking time to enjoy the baby and the importance of mutual enjoyment in interactions is stressed in informal conversations with the mothers. (Clark and Seifer found that asking mothers such questions as "Who do you remember having the most fun playing with when you were a child?", "How did that feel?", and "What is the most fun thing for you to do now?" helped mothers recall feelings of delight and playfulness.)

5. *Acknowledging.* In order to acknowledge a baby's particular behavior, a mother must notice that behavior and respond contingently with an appropriate gesture or vocalization. A fussy, difficult baby may frustrate a mother in her attempts to

acknowledge infant responses, especially if the infant's responses are not predictable or easily readable. Reviewing the videotapes makes it possible to identify specific behaviors that need to be acknowledged with a look of animation, a smile, or a verbal response. The mother is encouraged to notice how the frequency of the infant's behavior is affected by the contingency of parental behavior. At this level, special emphasis is placed on the exchange of appropriate emotions, since emotional signaling between infant and caregiver forms the basis for communicating needs, intentions, and satisfactions (Emde, 1988).

6. *Imitating.* Imitation of the baby is a very effective means of increasing maternal sensitivity. Mothers need to do more than just acknowledge their babies' behavior; they need to reinforce the babies' behavior in ways that promote reciprocal interaction and enhance the babies' sense of independence and self. Imitation not only improves mothers' observational skills; it also produces a feeling of excitement in the babies as they realize that their own behavior is directing the interaction.

A mother may be asked to imitate in different ways. First, she is asked not to talk to the baby, but to do everything that the baby does when there is eye contact. Next, she is asked to imitate only the baby's sounds. In reviewing the videotapes, particular attention is paid to the baby's sound production and affect during the interaction. Informal discussion focuses on the role vocal imitation (or any contingent verbal response) plays in turn taking, and on the importance of turn taking to language development. In addition, informal discussions about the importance of shared emotional experiences (begun in the preceding level) are continued.

7. *Elaborating and expanding.* Adolescent mothers usually look after their babies' physical needs, but often do not talk to their babies directly. A variety of strategies may be used to increase verbal interactions. A mother may be taught the following:

a. To expand on the baby's behavior by imitating that behavior and then chaining other behaviors to sustain the baby's interest. For example, the mother can clap her hands when the baby is clapping his or her hands, and can then vary the activity by playing "Pat-a-Cake." The game requires the mother to talk to the baby as she plays with him or her.

b. To talk to the baby, describing what the baby is doing or how he or she is feeling. For example:

> Oh, look at that smile, you must be happy.
> You really like that rattle.
> Oh, you dropped the rattle. Mommy will get it.
> Oh, look at your face, you're going to cry. You must be hungry. You want your bottle, don't you?
> You must have a tummyache. You need a burp.

c. To label the objects and actions in which she and her baby are jointly involved. During dressing, feeding, or bathing, the mother can label body parts and items of clothing, as well as the baby's movements. For example:

> You look warm. Let's take your sweater off. Pull out this arm, now this one. There, doesn't that feel better?
> Oh, your diaper is so wet, I'm going to change it. You're kicking your legs so fast. You really like not having that diaper on, don't you?
> Oh, you must be hungry, you're opening your mouth so wide. Here's your bottle.
> The water is warm. Here's ducky. Are you blowing bubbles?

Mothers are encouraged to speak in a slow, exaggerated manner; the content of the speech is not as important as the way in which it is delivered.

8. *Extended engaging.* This is the end point in the hierarchy, whereby parents are considered to demonstrate the most sensitive behavior. As defined by Clark and Seifer (1983), when a mother is routinely interacting with her infant at this level,

> she is aware of her child's signals of interest and fatigue, knows when to introduce new play activities, and is aware of the tempo her child needs to maintain a proper level of arousal. She reinforces and maintains infant behavior

through acknowledgment, imitation, elaboration, and expansion. In addition, the mother maintains interest through the timing and choice of new play behaviors. Most important, she is able to modify existing interaction patterns and engage in novel means of interaction with her baby. Conversely, the mothers do not force behavior on their bab[ies], nor do they inappropriately override baby behavior. (p. 80)

Although teaching mothers how to "play" with their infants appears deceptively simple, the intervention contains components that tap all developmental domains. Early mother–infant interaction is essential to the development of the interactive communication process (Kaye, 1982). Much of the initial acquisition of communication skills occurs as the mother and infant become finely attuned to each other through taking turns and acting reciprocally with each other during social play. A mother who fails to respond to the child's communications or who intrudes upon child-initiated activities distorts the interactive process (Stern, 1977), and disrupts the child's sense of competence in controlling his or her social environment (Watson, 1979, 1985; White, 1959). Failure to establish communication can have long-term detrimental effects on the child's development (Sameroff & Chandler, 1975). Social interactions are often limited, giving the child fewer opportunities to learn and to use communicative skills; this results in poor communicative abilities, which in turn may restrict cognitive development as well as social interaction with peers.

Improvements in the quality of interaction can lead to a self-perpetuating system of adaptive behavior. With intervention, mothers become more sensitive to their infants' cues; as a result, their infants become more skilled in communication and social interaction. In turn, increases in the infants' skills make the mothers more confident in their ability to engage the infants in interaction. The mothers feel more competent and experience greater self-esteem, which makes them even more effective parents. Interactions become more and more mutually satisfying, to the benefit of both parents and children.

TABLE 5.1. Methods for Enhancing Parental Sensitivity with Preschool-Age Children: An Overview of Training Objectives (arranged in approximate order of introduction)

Parent-focused objectives
1. Parents are connected to corollary services in the community that provide peer activities, social support, and child care assistance.
2. Parents learn to watch and follow the child's actions, without directing or interfering.
3. Parents learn to speak loudly and clearly, and to provide some narrative aloud of the child's ongoing activity.
4. Parents learn to display positive emotion spontaneously while watching and playing with their child, such as smiling, showing enthusiasm, and expressing interest in the child's activity.
5. Parents are taught to use verbal praise, hugs, and other positive reactions to the child's appropriate behavior.

Child-focused objectives
1. Special needs of the child are focused on during training exercises with parents, to improve on any weak areas of development.
2. The child is taught, via parental activities, to extend his or her attention span gradually.
3. The child's use of appropriate forms of communication, and expression of positive emotion, are taught during activities with parents.

Behaviors to minimize or avoid
1. Telling the child what to do or how to behave.
2. Emotionless expression or communication (facial, verbal, physical, etc.).
3. Harsh words, criticism, or commands.
4. Interfering with the child's activity.
5. The use of the word "No!"

Interventions that reflect developmental changes and vary in accordance with developmental level hold considerable promise as child abuse prevention strategies (Wekerle & Wolfe, 1991). However, the importance of related support services for families cannot be overshadowed by this optimism. Studies have shown perceived social support to be directly related to the quality of parent–infant interaction. Frequent contact with supportive health care professionals can have a positive effect on parental behavior (Crnic, Greenberg, Ragozin, Robinson, & Basham, 1983), as can living with supportive members of the extended family (Stevens, 1984). In conjunction with these and other community-based services to disadvantaged families, methods for enhancing early interactional skills through social play are nonthreatening and enjoyable ways to increase parental sensitivity and nurturing behavior. The benefits of such opportunities can be far-reaching: Not only does such training facilitate healthy parent–child relationships and optimal child development, but the presence of mutually satisfying interactions and a secure infant–mother attachment relationship may bolster both a parent's and a child's resiliency to stress and disadvantage.

Methods for Enhancing Parental Sensitivity: B. Preschool-Age Children

Table 5.1 provides an overview of the training objectives during the first phase of treatment for families with preschoolers. The table is intended as a reference guide to therapists for assessing progress and reviewing objectives throughout the program. Most of the objectives are aimed at parental behavior, reflecting the belief that parents serve as primary facilitators of children's development. Several child-focused objectives are introduced during this phase of the program as well, and they expand during the second phase (see Chapter 6). The table also provides a reminder of the types of behaviors and interactions that are *discouraged* during each phase (e.g., parents' telling the child what to do or how to behave), in an effort to keep the focus on the primary objectives.

General Description

In line with the stated goal of improving the quality of the parent–child relationship, parental sensitivity and responsivity to children form a primary focus of the program. Once a child is comfortable being alone with the therapist (this can take anywhere from a few minutes to several sessions), parents are asked to go and observe the interaction from behind a one-way mirror. We find that parents are more willing to engage in the program if they are not asked to participate very actively in the beginning, when they are most uncomfortable and self-conscious. Their expectation may be that the therapist will conduct the "work" with the child, and so this procedure meets with their initial expectations. The therapist asks parents simply to observe, and he or she places minimal restrictions or pressure on the child. This allows the therapist to interact more freely with the child, and more importantly serves to offer the child (and parents!) a period of low-key adjustment to this unfamiliar and somewhat threatening situation.

Parents may be surprised that they are not being asked to "do anything" at first other than watch. Our instructions to observe are couched in terms of the importance of the therapist's getting to know the child; consequently, parents usually are tolerant of this delay in receiving any immediate assistance. At the same time, the therapist may acknowledge for them their perceptions that their child can be difficult at times, and remind them that the most successful way to deal with such difficulty is through a gradual learning process that applies the things they will be taught to real problems at home.

During this startup period, the therapist models appropriate voice tone, volume, and clarity, as well as eye contact with the child, in an effort to encourage the parents to watch and enjoy what their young child does. The therapist *follows the child's lead,* rather than directing the child. Less emphasis is placed at this point on guidance of the child or management of disruptive or off-task situations (although the therapist may do so spontaneously as required). The parents need to develop an awareness of their child's own interests, style, and manner of communicating before more direction and expectations can be introduced. Such modeling is then rehearsed by parents over several sessions until the therapist and parents agree that the low-key situations can be maintained with the child, and that parents are attending to the child's ongoing behavior with appropriate (i.e., noncritical, enthusiastic) emotional, physical, and verbal responses.

The therapeutic purpose of this low-key, nonstressful therapist–child interaction is twofold. First of all, it allows children to adjust gradually to the situation and to the therapist, and also allows parents to adjust to the situation without being required to perform in any fashion. Second, we have found that this introduces parents to the importance of enjoying and playing with their children in a low-stress, spontaneous fashion. As others have also noted, many at-risk parents are uncomfortable simply playing with their children, and consequently turn a normal play situation into a more stressful compliance task for the children (e.g., Crittenden & Bonvillian, 1984; Oldershaw, Walters, & Hall, 1986). In addition, many parents seem somewhat surprised to discover that their children *can* play in a positive way without being destructive or disruptive. To put it simply, they have seldom experienced (or perceived) enjoyable interactions with their children. Observing a therapist and a child interacting with each other peacefully (or, at times, not so peacefully!) can provide parents with some encouragement and confirmation of their needs.

The materials used for this component of the program are typically simple toys (e.g., puppets, cars and trucks, coloring books, building blocks); the activities employed are ones that tap developmental level and skills (e.g., simple object identification games, counting tasks, sensory–motor activities, guessing games, etc.). The Pyramid Scales (Cone, 1984) or similar developmentally derived measures are particularly useful for providing meaningful activities with children that will keep them involved for 20 to 30 minutes. Throughout this period of time, the therapist speaks loudly and openly in the room, and the parents hear everything that is going on via microphones connected to a television monitor.

When observing behind the one-way mirror, parents are told to take particular note of the tone of voice used by the therapist; the types of questions or guidance provided to the child; the use of props, cues, or signals by the therapist to assist the child; and any use of "control techniques" by the therapist to reduce distraction or difficult behavior. Once they are familiar with this arrangement, parents are given a notepad and pen to write down their observations; this enables them to act as the "impartial observers" for a while.

Whenever a therapist feels that he or she is not achieving the intended purpose with a child, the therapist states such a feeling openly and candidly in the room for the parents to hear. In this manner parents see that these feelings are normal, and that they can be managed more easily if one identifies them early rather than attempting to hide them. If the child grows tired or the task becomes too difficult, the therapist again states this observation for parents to hear, and then shifts to another activity or ends the session.

After two or three sessions of such observation and developmental stimulation on the part of the therapist, parents are ready to participate in these "warmup exercises." We often structure the situation at first by providing some appropriate toys and activities, or asking parents to bring in their own materials. The instructions given to the parents simply state that they are to enjoy some time with the child, and to make observations about what they see the child doing. They are discouraged from using too much guidance with the child, but rather are directed simply to observe and verbally note any observations or thoughts, which the therapist can hear.

At the end of 10 or 15 minutes, we interrupt the session to ask parents for any observations or feelings they may have about what has been going on. In particular, we are interested in their observations of the child; we wish to determine whether they are sensitive to their child's *normal behavior* under these optimal conditions. At the same time, we do not hide our realization that things will be more difficult under "battle conditions" at home during stressful periods. Parents are assured that these low-stress interactions will go a long way in reducing the attention-seeking behaviors of their child later on.

Rehearsal and feedback of the basic skills of attending to normal child activity are crucial aspects of all phases of the program. Parents must receive accurate and honest feedback regarding their progress, but this feedback must be couched in terms that are not too harsh or that would lead to defensiveness. One technique that is quite effective in this regard is to allow time at the end of each session to view parts of the preceding videotape; this permits the parents (and the child, if old enough) to see their own interactions and to comment on their behavior. In most cases the child is entertained by a staff member while the parents and therapist view this tape alone. Parents are encouraged to use their own descriptive terms or labels when describing interactions with their child; this limits the use of terms that are unfamiliar or poorly understood.

Typically, parents often enjoy this phase of training. Somewhat to our surprise, they have little difficulty criticizing their own behavior with their children if they are permitted to do so nonjudgmentally. This is a particularly valuable aspect of the training, for it allows the therapist to determine how parents view their own behavior and how critical they are of themselves. Parents who themselves were raised in a highly critical and abusive home will be quite blunt in describing their own harsh parenting style, even though they may not view this style as being the cause of family problems. As expected, such harshness is visible during interactions with their child. As parents become more alert to their own style and are able to criticize its weaknesses and choose alternatives, the parent–child relationship begins to reflect this positive change through spontaneous positive emotion, improved child attention, and decreased negativism.

Some Clinical Illustrations

To accomplish the principal objectives of this first intervention phase (see Table 5.1), we have relied on several simple approaches for encouraging parents to try out unfamiliar activities with their children. In the first type of situation illustrated below, parents are unfamiliar with the new tasks or interactions; yet they seem relatively interested in trying, once the procedure is carefully explained and modeled for them. (In our experience, such parents account for a slight majority of our clients.) Typical comments or actions that a therapist may model for parents are shown first, followed by illustrative therapist comments and actions.

In the second type of situation, parents are less engaged, are more resistant or uncomfortable in the situation, or require more concrete assistance during this phase. The examples of therapist interactions and comments focus especially on parental lack of emotional responsivity to the child (parent-focused objectives 3, 4, and 5 in Table 5.1), beause this is often a major problem for resistant clients.

The third type of situation centers more closely on child-focused objectives. In the examples provided here, the children are developmentally delayed or behaviorally difficult to engage in the intended activities. Suggestions for improving basic communication prerequisites and establishing the basis for parental guidance are provided.

SITUATION 1: INTERESTED PARENTS; RELATIVELY TYPICAL CHILD

In the first type of situation, the therapist begins by modeling play interactions with the child, while the parents observe. Then each parent is asked to take a turn with the child. The emphasis is initially upon passive observation and commentary regarding the child's activity (objective 2). During subsequent sessions, the therapist encourages each parent to be spontaneous, and to show enthusiasm and praise in response to the child's ongoing activity (objectives 3, 4, & 5). The therapist may initiate interaction with the child as follows:

> Hi, Jimmy! Let's find a new toy in here and see what we can do with it. Look! You found how to make it squeak and whistle *(pauses and observes for several seconds)*. You can make the train move and make noises *(pause)*. Now you are is picking up the doll and touching its hair. Is the hair soft? You are smiling at the doll. The doll's eyes close when it's put to sleep. You are patting the doll and putting it to bed.

The child may turn to a new activity, and the therapist follows:

> What is that you are playing with? The doll has a teddy bear, just like your own! The bear is brown, with big dark eyes. You are touching his [eyes, ears, nose, etc.].

Similar commentary and observation continues for 10–15 minutes. If the child shows fatigue or distress, the therapist can offer a break and change:

> I think it's time to take a break for a snack, and then have Mommy come in and play for a while. Can you show her what you have in here? I'll bet she'd like to see some of your toys!

A parent is then led into the room, and the therapist may sit in the background or behind the one-way mirror. The parent is told:

> See if you can watch what Jimmy is doing and follow along, commenting on whatever you notice. There's no need at this point to choose things for him; rather, just watch, listen, and talk to him as he plays.

Following such modeling and rehearsal opportunities, the therapist has the parents observe video segments, to encourage their own comments and to provide constructive feedback for the next session:

> Let's go look at the tape of what you've been doing. I'd like you to tell me anything you can about what you were thinking and feeling during the session, and how you think Jimmy felt. We'll stop the tape whenever you'd like to discuss something.

In lieu of videotaped segments, the therapist and parents can discuss particular things that were happening:

> Remember when Jimmy was playing with the teddy bear? What were you thinking and feeling at that time?

The therapist provides mild feedback to each parent, pointing out first his or her *appropriate* behaviors during the interaction. Areas in need of improvement are noted in a positive manner, avoiding any implication of inadequacy or criticism:

> You were *very good* at following Jimmy's behavior and letting him play comfortably. I noticed that you looked him in the eyes when speaking, and that your words were clear and easy to understand. That's really important for young children, because they need to know you're paying attention, and they need to hear things as clearly as possible.
>
> I also noticed that you showed a great deal of interest in Jimmy's activity, by being enthusiastic ("Wow—you put the pieces of the puzzle together yourself!") and by avoiding any criticism if he lost interest momentarily. Next time I think we'll try a situation where you can show Jimmy how you feel by giving him a hug, or telling him how good he has been while playing.

SITUATION 2: UNCOMFORTABLE PARENTS; RELATIVELY TYPICAL CHILD

In the second type of situation, one or both parents are very cautious and seemingly uncomfortable playing with the child in the manner shown by the therapist. Such a parent looks at the child, but his or her words lack any enthusiasm and fail to convey interest or involvement in the activity. The child plays independently, almost as if the parent were not in the room. At the same time, the parent says and does little with the child, as if to avoid any possible disruption or annoyance.

When a parent is very overcontrolled and wary, the major objective is to help him or her to relax and enjoy some time with their child. This can be accomplished in the most straightforward manner by keeping the activities and instructions very simple and brief, and gradually building more confidence and spontaneity. The therapist aims at first only to have parent and child play together side by side, without requiring any "action" on the part of the parent until he or she is more comfortable. The parent is encouraged to use nonverbal interactions with the child, and is instructed to "see if you can help Jimmy have a fun time with the toys for a few minutes." The therapist avoids "pressuring" or "correcting" the parent, for this will probably produce more apathy and withdrawal.

Sessions may be reduced in length, or broken up by more therapist involvement with the child, to permit a gradual acclimatization to the unfamiliar (and perhaps threatening) situation for such a parent. The therapist must be sensitive to each parent's individual approach or style with his or her child, in an attempt to avoid undermining the parent's own unique style and characteristics.

The following illustration begins at the point where a parent is asked to come into the playroom and play with the child. The therapist says to the parent:

> What makes Tom laugh and smile? Is there a game the two of you like to play that he really enjoys? I'd like to see what Tom's like when he's having a great time. He seems a bit shy and quiet this morning, so let's find a fun game and let him "settle in" for a while. If there's anything you would normally do at home to have fun with him, please feel free to do it here!

If the parent speaks too softly and hesitantly, or the child shows little interest in playing with the parent, the therapist may join in the activity on the floor. The therapist may direct the child to an activity that requires some parental participation. The therapist may remain in the room to keep the "mood" of the interactions light and enjoyable, and to counter a somber or serious atmosphere with humor.

> Look how Tom piles all of the farm animals into the barn. They'll never get to sleep with all that racket! Tom has a terrific smile when he's having a good time—is he like this much of the time? I noticed that he starts to laugh whenever you pick up one of the

> animals. I think he really wants you to show him where
> they go.

Brief videotaped or recalled excerpts are then used to review the interchange and discuss parental feelings about the treatment methods. This provides important opportunities to pinpoint parental dissatisfaction or discomfort early on, so that adjustments can be made.

> Well, what do you think? I'd be interested in knowing
> what you were thinking about during this activity
> [being reviewed on tape].

If a parent seems reluctant to volunteer a feeling or opinion, the therapist can offer a remark to "get things started":

> I think Tom's a pretty active guy, who probably tries to
> get away with a bit too much when you let him play
> with whatever he'd like. Does that happen at home?

During subsequent sessions, once a parent is more comfortable and willing to play spontaneously, the therapist introduces more comments to elicit parental self-feedback regarding emotional tone and reactions to the child. An attempt is made to direct more of the parent's attention to the child's positive and desirable behaviors, no matter how small, and away from surveillance and control:

> I'm glad you noticed when Tom was playing quietly
> just then. You had asked him to quit throwing things,
> and you thanked him when he did. While watching the
> tape, tell me *each time* you come to a spot where you felt
> pleased with what was going on. Also, tell me *each time*
> you were upset, with either Tom or yourself.

The following exercise is particularly useful for identifying sensitive issues for a parent. Some parents are overly harsh on themselves; some are overly harsh on the children; and some are both. We spend as much time as is necessary to review these situations, and perhaps elicit new examples for recording, in order to gain a full understanding of the patterns that precede a negative encounter at home. Although we do not role-play a parent's *negative* side (because this would be too threatening), we may demonstrate for the parent how to express feelings of ambivalence, annoyance, or confusion openly while involved in an activity with the child. As the parent observes, the therapist may say:

> Tom seems to be wound up today. I hope I can get him to find something interesting to do. Uh-oh, looks like he doesn't want to play with the farm. Let's put that one away and try something else. (*Child starts to cry.*) I'm not sure what I've done, but Tom's upset. Maybe he's a bit scared being here without Mom, so I think I'll comfort him. (*Child screams louder and won't allow contact.*) He's probably upset because we put the toy away, but I don't think it's a good idea to give in to that. So let's switch to a new activity, or take a break. Sometimes you just can't expect to figure out what kids are up to, so you just do the best you can. Sometimes my 4-year-old does this, and I get a bit annoyed. Usually the situation stops once we calm ourselves down and look for a new activity.

SITUATION 3: CONFUSED PARENTS;
UNUSUALLY CHALLENGING CHILD

In any program involved with dysfunctional families, parents are only half of the picture; considerable attention must be given to the individual needs and challenges that the children provide. This program offers flexibility not only in allowing a child to adjust to the unfamiliar situations; more importantly, we attempt to tailor the activities early on to the particular strengths and weaknesses of each child.

As shown in the examples below, we select activities that will maximize a child's attention, and that provide ample opportunity for pleasant interchanges during the initial sessions.

Often children present initially as withdrawn, fearful, or overactive. Some children show signs of developmental delay, such as speech and language delay, poor attention span, and little eye contact. Although these delays and behavior problems are addressed more specifically during subsequent sessions (see Chapter 6), at this point we are interested primarily in setting the stage for improved attention and learning in sessions to follow. The approach relies heavily on ongoing therapist commentary regarding the child's feelings, behavior, and activities, in an attempt to settle the child and encourage parental focus on these "prelearning" skills.

In some cases, a child may show little interest in activities and may withdraw from the therapist. New games are looked at only briefly, then discarded. The therapist may say:

> Sally, look at how I build a tower with the blocks! Would you like to try? *(Therapist hands a block to child; she throws it down.)* Oh, well, let's find the puppet. *(Therapist talks to Sally with puppet, getting her to show some emotion. Then, aloud for parents to hear:)* Sally is not sure what we're doing today, but I think she likes the puppet to speak. I'm looking for things that catch her eye, and trying to show her a lot of positive expression and enthusiasm, to ease her worries and make her more comfortable.

In other cases, a child may have very limited speech, and may communicate with noises and tugs at the therapist. The therapist listens for sounds that can be repeated with meaning (e.g., "mine," "doggy"), and responds with verbal commentary and positive emotion to the child's attempts to communicate:

> You would like to play with the truck, Billy? Can you say "truck" for me? Good try! Let's pick it up and have it make noises. Look at me, Billy—t-, t-, t-, truck! Good! *(Billy grabs therapist sharply.)* What do you want to do? Show me. I think you want to get the blocks out to play. Say "block!" OK, let's dump them out!

Often, a child will show a very limited attention span and will try to run around the room. In this case, the therapist finds one or two highly engaging activities, such as sound-producing games and puppets, and draws the child's attention to this game. As soon as the child starts to lose interest, the therapist switches to a new activity briefly. All other distractions are removed from the room. The child is not physically restrained from walking away, but rather is drawn back by the change in activity. If this proves unsuccessful, a break is given, and the activity is started again afterwards.

> You like to explore everything, don't you, John? Look! I have a talking doll! Can you make him say something? Excellent—he spoke to you! (*John starts to go for toy chest.*) Look, John! I have a puppet. Would you like to hold him? Good, you're coming back to play with me. After we play with the puppet, Mommy will come in and play too! When we're all done, we'll go have a snack. Can you stack these blocks? Oops, you knocked them down—that looked like fun. Let's try again, only this time you put one on here for me.

The therapist closely guides the child in this instance, since he is not finding things to do on his own and is becoming too distracted.

Upon completion of these activities with the child, the therapist and parents review the tape. This time the focus is on what *the child* may have been feeling, thinking, and so forth; and the therapist uses the difficult situations to express empathy with the parents for the "challenge that kids can be at times." The parents are told of the strategy to keep their child on task for longer and longer periods of time (from a few seconds to a few minutes), and are cautioned not to expect anything further for a while. The therapist provides a specific activity to practice (e.g., reading a story), and tells the parents to look for ways of spending a few uninterrupted minutes several times a day with the child to increase his or her attention span.

In sum, the initial phase of intervention may be relatively short for some families (i.e., if both parents and children fulfill the objectives easily), or it may extend for some time, in an effort to improve on parents' responsivity to the children, and/or on the children's basic developmental needs. Once these foundations have been adequately established, the program moves on to increase appropriate parental demands and directions for the children.

6

Intervention: II. Methods for Improving Parental Teaching, Discipline, and Anger Management

As parents and children begin to form a more positive relationship, we introduce additional exercises aimed at child stimulation, improved child compliance, and more effective parental discipline. "Child compliance" and "parental discipline" are relative terms, whose meanings depend partially on what parents are willing and able to teach and enforce (and, of course, the child's activity level, attention span, and similar developmental competence). Thus, we set no specific goal for levels of child compliance or parental discipline per se; rather, we view compliance as an important vehicle for teaching parents to use appropriate commands, guidance, and teaching strategies.

By this point, most parents are anxious to learn more about "control methods." They may have been officially told to give up the typical control methods they have been using at home (i.e., physical punishment; harsh verbal criticism or berating), and are often feeling frustrated by their children's growing noncompliance and difficult behavior. The transition to this important aspect of training, however, can be straightforward once parents have seen some benefits of increasing positive attention with their children.

In practice, helping parents to gain more child cooperation and compliance is often taught along with corresponding disciplinary practices. Controlling their own anger and arousal, while simultaneously attempting to manage or discipline a young, distraught child, clearly poses a major challenge to *all* parents. For this important reason, we begin our training of parents in effective discipline methods by discussing with them the purpose of discipline, its limits and forms, and its pitfalls. For clinical purposes, the following procedures are not intended to be applied in a rigid manner, or necessarily in the order we have presented. Rather, this presentation highlights the major training objectives and procedures for improving parental stimulation and disciplinary methods, and provides examples along the way of how the material can build on skills already developed. Depending on the needs of each family, and the family's commitment to training at this point in the program, a therapist may choose to introduce disciplinary methods at an earlier point in time.

Setting Reasonable Expectations for Children's Emotional and Behavioral Development

Table 6.1 provides an overview of training objectives designed to improve how parents teach developmentally relevant skills to their preschool-age children, and to teach parents to set reasonable limits for child compliance. These teaching and limit-setting abilities establish the necessary foundation for applying discipline in a fair and effective manner. Training principally consists of two interrelated components: (1) exercises aimed at stimulating several areas of child development (an extension of some of the techniques described in Chapter 5); and (2) discussion of parental expectations for children, with training in limit setting and appropriate commands. At this point the program turns more towards boosting the parents' important role as teachers and guides for their children, and parents learn how to approach this role with more confidence. In close conjunction with this training, we then begin to introduce effective discipline

TABLE 6.1. Setting Reasonable Expectations for Children's Emotional and Behavioral Development: An Overview of Training Objectives (arranged in approximate order of introduction)

Parent-focused objectives

1. Parents are taught activities to promote child's language and interpersonal skills development
2. Parents review their child expectations with therapist, and work at defining and setting appropriate limits and expectations
3. Parents learn to use verbal guidance and proper commands with child, when attempting to teach child or to limit child's off-task behavior
4. Parents learn to use unambiguous, appropriate expressions of affect when giving commands, monitoring compliance or activities of the child, and when administering praise and expressing interest.

Child-focused objectives

1. The child learns to attend to tasks and activities for longer periods of time, and begins to display an enthusism for learning and playing.
2. The child learns to comply more often to parental requests, in accordance with his or her level of development and (modified) parental expectations.
3. The child gradually strengthens any developmental weaknesses in communication and social interaction.

---

strategies and coping techniques aimed at addressing current problems and typical child-related aggravations (this topic is dealt with in a later section of the chapter).

Promoting Child Development and Adaptive Behavior

The training procedures supporting the goal of balancing parental sensitivity and demandingness are linked closely with the promotion of children's adaptive behavior. There is considerable evidence, as cited in Chapter 2, that infant and child characteristics can affect the probability of abuse. Such characteristics may be mental, physical, or behavioral abnormalities present from birth, or may be learned behaviors that increase the likelihood of abuse, such as negative attention seeking, noncompliance, or screaming. Although the cause–effect relationship is not clear, efforts directed at remediating maladaptive or deficient developmental patterns can serve to benefit both positive parent–child interactions and child development.

This developmental component also serves to make training more relevant and attractive, especially to parents with preschool-age children, who often are challenging because of their emerging but incomplete developmental competencies. Training initially continues to be aimed at increasing the positive nature of parent–child interactions (e.g., positive physical contact, positive child experiences, nonaversive control). Gradually, parents are shown through modeling, role playing, and feedback how to choose and engage in daily activities with their children that serve to strengthen the children's areas of deficiency and to promote adaptive functioning.

Specific areas of functioning most relevant to the prevention of emotional and physical maltreatment include children's verbal and social abilities. Although a large proportion of children with delayed speech and language development at 3 years of age may catch up, such delays may in turn lead to further delays in other critical areas. The "teaching style" of many parents referred for early intervention in our program is far less explicit and less effective than that of more advantaged parents. Similarly, their children exhibit cognitive and behavioral deficits that often seem to perpetuate social rejection and inattention from others.

In regard to remediating these developmental deficits and maladaptive responses of some abused children, the most important thing to keep in mind is that favorable adult responses are associated with increases in positive child behaviors. Positive child behaviors include expressions of positive affect, moderate activity level, responsiveness to adult interactions and feedback, and age-appropriate language and social skills. Thus, our strategy is to enhance the developmental and adaptive abilities of each child, in conjunction with positive child-rearing objectives for each parent.

We select specific activities that are aimed at the development of age-appropriate language abilities (e.g., eye contact, responding to simple sounds or phrases, producing sounds, etc.) and social interaction skills (e.g., following directions, engaging in play with parents, expressing affection and needs). In many cases these activities are self-evident, such as having parents emphasize certain sounds more clearly or practice a simple command (e.g., "Look at me"). We also refer children for a developmental screening assessment whenever more specific concerns or delays are suspected.

In addition, we increase the degree of flexibility at this stage, to allow for the developmental needs of each child. For families with younger children, more time is spent on identifying and reinforcing the toddlers' attending to the parents, uttering speech-like sounds, and making efforts to comply with simple commands (e.g., "Go get the ball and roll it to me, please"). The goal is to increase both the quantity and the quality of positive parent–child interactions; thus, there is less emphasis with very young children on discipline or punishment techniques. Preschoolers receive a greater emphasis on furthering their language development and social interaction skills. Several suggestions for specific activities to promote child development and adaptive behavior are given in Table 6.2.

Setting Reasonable Expectations for Child Compliance

Compliance is considered to be a critical accomplishment in establishing positive interactions between parents and children. From studies of how competent parents interact with their children, researchers have learned that such parents closely monitor the children's state of attention or involvement, and adapt the nature of their requests according to this state (Maccoby & Martin, 1983). Although we should not expect such "ideal" (perhaps unrealistic) planning and follow-through with at-risk parents, it is worthwhile to explain the advantages of ensuring that a child is oriented to a parent before compliance is expected. If the child is engrossed in play or some high-interest activity, for example, the parent should expect to orient the child prior to

TABLE 6.2. Examples of Activities to Promote Child Development and Adaptive Behavior

---

Speech and language
- Identify objects in the playroom that the child can pronounce or approximate. Make a fuss over the child for identifying and pronouncing these objects during clinic visits. For toddlers, encourage and repeat sounds that are easy for them to make and can be connected to actual objects or people, (e.g., "'ba' is for 'ball'—Sally has the ball").
- Play a game in which the child is told to find something beginning with a certain sound ("Can you find something in this room that begins with 'T,' like in 'Tommy'?"). Each time the child locates something with that sound, he or she pronounces the sound and is praised for making an effort.
- Encourage the child to attempt pronunciations for each and every request; model and rehearse difficult pronunciations without correcting or criticizing the child's sounds.
- Sing songs and read stories at every chance!
- Repeat sounds and words that the child emits, letting her know that you are pleased with his or her efforts to make the proper sounds ("Train! That's right! The *train* is coming!").

Sensory–motor and social interactional skills
- Use building blocks and similar assembly toys to have the child make his or her own creations.
- Engage child in physically active play (e.g., tickling, rolling over, running, climbing, leapfrog).
- Play simple games that require the child to take turns, pass objects, or participate actively (e.g., puzzles, tic-tac-toe, bingo).
- Dance and play musical instruments.
- Play imaginary games that involve the child's favorite characters or activities (e.g., hide and seek).
- Play "follow the leader" and "Simple Simon" games that encourage attention, compliance, and imagination.
- Have child imitate different facial expressions (of happiness, anger, fear, silliness, etc.), to encourage imagination and to provide paractice in following simple directions.

---

issuing a command. The initial statement from the parent may be one of orientation (e.g., "Let me see what you're playing with"), followed soon thereafter with instructions to begin putting away the toys.

Several of the objectives noted in Table 6.1 are designed to improve parental respect for the child's own competence and individuality, which plays a critical role in developing a healthy parent–child relationship. Parents who are themselves cooperative and attentive to their children's needs and capabilities tend to have children who are similarly cooperative and easier to manage. In contrast, parents who rely on intrusive and power-assertive methods of control are likely to have offspring who respond in kind with annoying and disruptive behavior.

In practical terms, the teaching of appropriate parental commands and directions designed to elicit child compliance should begin with a review and discussion of parental expectations and "implicit rules." Many at-risk parents ascribe greater negative intentionality to their children's behavior than do low-risk parents (Larrance & Twentyman, 1984), and also have more unrealistic expectations of what is appropriate to expect from their child (Azar & Rohrbeck, 1986). Thus, parents are encouraged to express their views openly about what they believe their child is up to, or why the child is doing (or not doing) what he or she is asked to do. An active approach to eliciting parental cognitions about children is necessary, because exercises aimed at eliciting thoughts and feelings are often difficult at first.

One of the most effective ways of eliciting parents' current thoughts and feelings is to review a recent problem they have had with their child. Once parents have described the scene in vivid detail, the therapist can ask what they would be saying to themselves at that moment, and how that statement might affect their actions. Questioning parents about a recent annoyance involving the child typically begins by having them simply state their feelings. Then they are asked why the child's behavior made them feel that way, or what the parents expected of the child in the situation (Azar & Wolfe, 1989). It may be helpful to link these feelings to any other interpersonal situations, such as arguments with a spouse, relative, or employer:

Are there any other times when you feel this way? Do any other individuals make you feel this way sometimes?

The therapist can facilitate this exercise by falling back on his or her own examples and experiences with children, especially when interacting with the child while the parent watches. Whenever the child fails to comply, or is disruptive, the therapist can express aloud his or her feelings:

> I'm not sure just what to do yet—Jane seems to be uninterested in listening at the moment. Rather than getting angry, I think I'll wait a minute or two and try again. I've seen my 3-year-old do this, and I know you can't always expect kids to listen.

Parents who lack basic familiarity with young children can be exposed to their habits, abilities, and demands by being given opportunities to observe children under less stressful circumstances. The peer support group can play an active role here: The other members' children can be observed by parents (usually in pairs), with a therapist or teacher who can point out things to notice. Parents can be given simple challenges, such as having them guess what will happen when the children are required to put the toys away, to focus on a less interesting task, and so on. Parents are encouraged to enjoy the humorous side of parenting, and to be sensitive to the limitations, communication styles, and demandingness of young children. Observing children from a distance not only removes some of the pressure on parents to play the "parent role," but also serves to desensitize them to the noise and activity level to which they will be expected to adapt at home as their children grow older. Exposure to other children who are engaged in different activities, therefore, may go a long way in providing parents with a standard of normal behavior for their own children, and in suggesting to them how to respond or not to respond to such behavior.

Teaching parents how to improve their child's compliance to their requests follows closely from the programs developed by Forehand and McMahon (1981) and others. We begin with a structured and simple compliance task, in order to reinforce the child's compliance and to teach appropriate verbal commands to the parents. Once again, this component begins by having the therapist model appropriate commands while the parents observe behind the one-way mirror. Depending on the age of the child, most often this task involves very simple commands that the child can easily comply with, such as rolling a ball back to the therapist, putting pegs in the hole, and so forth. The goal is to work up to more difficult compliance situations, such as picking up toys or following parental directions under distracting circumstances, which are introduced soon thereafter, along with discipline techniques (see following section). To achieve this goal, the parents need to understand the importance of using clear commands and following through with stated consequences.

The therapist may then request the child to do something more challenging and less interesting, such as putting away desired toys. He or she models for parents appropriate voice level, clarity of the request, and proper emotional tone to fit the request. Parents are instructed to repeat the command once, and then to repeat it again, adding a consequence for noncompliance after the third request (of course, if the child is not attending, or the circumstances are too distracting, parents are told to deal with these issues first). Once again, this skill is taught gradually by beginning with very simple requests and very minor consequences. For example, the child is told to pick up the toys; if he or she does not respond, the therapist models how to repeat this command, adding the consequence of some minor loss of privilege if the child does not comply:

> It's now time to start cleaning up, Jimmy. I'll put the blocks away while you put the cars and trucks in the box. If we get this done quickly, we can go and watch the TV pictures like we did last time! (*If child does not comply, but is attending:*) Please pick up the toys now. (*Therapist waits and observes; if child moves to comply in any fashion, he or she is praised and assisted. If there is no attempt, therapist states:*) Pick up the toys right now, or we can't go and watch the TV pictures of you and Mommy.

If the situation results in little compliance or attention on the part of a child, or if it raises a sense of frustration or upset on the part of either a parent or a child, the therapist should return to a simpler, more manageable task. Parents and children should not be pushed too quickly to achieve desired changes, because this poses the risk of failure and disillusionment. Rather, parents should be made aware of the fact that children will not always comply, and sometimes a parent has to decide either to follow through on a consequence (if one has been stated), or to abandon the attempt.

Compliance training can lead to disruptive behavior on the part of the child. Rather than seeing this as a cause of concern, we welcome such opportunities in order to model for parents how to respond to and cope with such typical events. We approach this in a lighthearted fashion, often repeating (so that the parents can hear) our recognition that the child is "perhaps too interested in the activity to listen at this time" or other coping statements aimed at helping parents to recognize that no one holds the key to getting children to listen or comply every time. Because many of us have children of our own, we may also point out some of the circumstances that remind us of how our own children behave at times. We feel it is important for clients to see that their children are not necessarily different from other children, and that even the "experts" do not expect or receive compliance all of the time.

Parents are told to pay particular attention to how the therapist uses commands, consequences, and praise to match the child's flow of behavior. Afterwards, parents are asked to identify and assert what they believe to be their own most natural, comfortable, and effective manner of responding to child noncompliance. The therapists must make every effort to preserve and respect this individual style throughout the remainder of training, allowing parents to monitor and critique the positives and negatives of their approach continuously. Of course, if the style is overly harsh, inconsistent, or inappropriate in some fashion, the therapist gradually (and tactfully!) adds suggestions for a parent to try during the next interaction:

> Mary, you really do a great job of watching Betsy to see if she follows through on your request. It's important that parents let their kids know that they are paying close attention, so I think your style is terrific in terms of her need for supervision and guidance. Do you think Betsy is relaxed and at ease when you ask her to do

something? *(Parent acknowledges child's overconcern with watching parent, perhaps out of fear.)* Is there anything we might try to help her relax? I notice that you enjoy playing music for her, so why don't you tell her that as soon as she's [completed the request], you'll play the kazoo with her? I think she'll feel more at ease knowing that you plan to do something fun right away.

During compliance training, the therapist also uses every opportunity to model appropriate parental affect. When dismayed or concerned about the child's misbehavior, the therapist uses appropriate facial expression, firmer voice tone, and other cues to communicate clearly to the child disapproval of his or her behavior (without frightening or confusing the child). Conversely, when the child is attempting to comply, the therapist will model appropriate positive affect (smiles, hugs, other forms of physical affection, and praise). Often parents need few verbal reminders to use such clear, unambiguous affective expressions; simply seeing over and over how the therapist shifts from being friendly to being firm to reinforcing the child's attempts influences their style in important ways.

Compliance training typically involves 10–15 minutes of the parents' observing the therapist with the child, followed by the therapists' observing each parent. Parents are encouraged to practice the same activities that the therapist has been doing with the child, and to speak openly about their frustration, annoyance, or pleasure at the child's reactions to commands. At this point, we often choose to use the "bug in the ear"—a microtransmitter that a parent can wear on his or her ear, in order to listen to the therapist from the observation room. We have found this to be particularly useful in situations in which a child poses quite a challenge to the parents, and parents need to be reminded how to focus on one command at a time. When using this device, the therapist provides minimal prompts only when necessary, but encourages the parent to speak openly and even to ask questions or express concerns throughout the interaction. This device also permits the therapist to reinforce parents immediately for improvements in their affect or command clarity, which has the added benefit of shaping this new behavior more quickly and readily. This device is not always needed, especially in situations where a child is old enough to be distracted by such a device, or in which a parent is uncomfortable using such a device. Nevertheless, it is quite helpful for short periods of time if a parent feels bewildered or confused as to how to engage the child in the task at hand.

At the close of each session, parents are again encouraged to view excerpts from their own interactions with the child for feedback purposes. They are encouraged to describe their performance in their own words, and to ask questions or seek further advice as to how to respond in the future. The therapist may choose to point out to parents any gains that are noticed from the previous session, as well as any need for improvements in particular areas of expression. Having the videotape in front of them makes it easier for parents to understand such feedback and to acknowledge its importance.

Clinical Illustration

We discovered the value of modeling how to handle failure during a compliance situation, which turned out to be an important clinical example that led to modifications in our training program. A 3-year-old boy, Timmy, was growing tired of the task he was being asked to complete by the therapist. Unaware that his mother was watching, and believing that he had the freedom to do what he wanted in the room, Timmy began to pick up toys and toss them, and to turn the light switch off and on. The therapist misjudged the situation, believing he could get Timmy under control without further incident. The therapist went to the chair that Timmy was standing on to reach the light switch, pulled him away, and brought him to the couch. At this point, Timmy went into a full temper tantrum and screamed violently while kicking and flailing his arms and legs.

The therapist attempted to talk over the noise Timmy was making so that his mother could hear his frustration and coping statements. However, Timmy's mother found the situation quite humorous and very familiar to her. A cotherapist, who was observing behind the mirror with the mother, noted that she expressed satisfaction in having Timmy's difficult behavior recognized by the therapist "firsthand." The cotherapist encouraged the mother to recognize that this was not a "trait" of Timmy, but rather a characteristic of most children of his age. In lighthearted "defense" of the therapist in the room, the mother was told that there is usually no easy solution for handling such a difficult situation. Rather, it was important only that the "parent" in this case maintain his composure and not expect to regain the child's compliance or cooperation at that point.

From this and many other unplanned "misadventures," we have learned that the spontaneous emergence of familiar problems during therapists' interactions with children adds authenticity to our program for parents (and, conveniently, often cannot be avoided!). Because a therapists' credibility can be difficult to establish (due to parent–therapist differences in education, lifestyle, etc.), such real-life events can serve to make the therapist more approachable and personable to parents. We use such events as opportunities to explain that a person cannot always expect to resolve a difficult situation to everyone's satisfaction. In such circumstances, parents (and therapists) can strive only to emerge from the situation as calmly as possible. When similar situations emerge during the course of treatment, therefore, therapists often will model the frustration and annoyance that they may feel, and parents are encouraged subsequently to talk about their own reactions under similar circumstances. Follow-up to these reactions is then added during the anger training phase of the program.

Teaching Anger Control and Effective Discipline Strategies

Teaching parents how to discipline their children effectively without resorting to physical or psychological threats or violent actions always poses unique and unforeseen challenges. It would be foolhardy to assume that our methods of discipline are the "correct" ones for all circumstances, and in fact we must go out of our way to provide information on discipline in a manner that is somewhat in keeping with each parent's views. To most parents,

TABLE 6.3. Anger Control and Effective Discipline Strategies: An Overview of Training Objectives (arranged in approximate order of introduction)

Parent-focused objectives

1. Parents learn to handle minor frustrations and setbacks with the child, by using humor, distraction, meaningful activities, and simple coping statements.
2. Parents begin to apply some basic skills to ongoing problems they have identified with their child.
3. Parents identify sources of anger and its self-expression, and learn to control arousal prior to disciplining the child.
4. Parents understand the "rules of punishment" and clarify their expectations for its short- and long-range impact.
5. Parents learn to use nonphysical, behavior-focused alternatives to corporal punishment, verbal coercion, or emotional abuse.
6. Parents practice anger control and appropriate discipline while engaging in live, provocative situations with their child.

Child-focused objectives

1. The child learns to respond to noncoercive, nonviolent discipline methods without escalating conflict.
2. The child reduces the frequency and intensity of major emotional outbursts or problem behaviors.

---

child discipline carries with it freedom of choice, family privacy, and fundamental rights of the individual. Moreover, they will remain unconvinced that other forms of discipline are better than their current ones unless they are closely involved in the effort to find an alternative approach.

Approaching the Topic with Parents

In recognition of the values associated with disciplinary choices, as well as the reality that no one technique is effective for everyone, we approach this topic in as nonauthoritarian, nonthreatening a manner as possible. Our goal is to help parents find a comfortable, preferred approach to punishment that offers the fewest negative risks to their children. We then assist parents in applying their preferred methods as appropriately and realistically as is feasible. One could argue, on the one hand, that parents who are at risk of emotional or physical abuse should be restricted entirely to nonphysical methods of discipline. On the other hand, parents will be more likely to continue using only those new methods that "fit" their own style and preferences, and only as long as they are generally effective. Clearly, one method of punishment or one strategy of discipline cannot apply to all parents. Primarily for this reason, our objectives and procedures are designed to be flexible in their application and modification. Table 6.3 provides an overview of our objectives.

To introduce this topic, we discuss what has usually been on the parents' mind since the beginning: "How do I control my child if I'm told I can't use physical punishment? I'm trying to make him [or her] mind me, just the same as my parents did!" To defuse the anxiety and defensiveness centered around the important and controversial topic of discipline, we first spend some time talking with parents about normal versus severe parenting practices. (We also find that parents are more attentive to this discussion after having spent some time with the therapist during the first phase of the intervention.) We introduce the topic of discipline by asking them to describe the extreme end points, from very harsh to very lenient. It is useful to place this description in the context of child maltreatment by asking how they define "child abuse," how they define "spoiling" of children, and what they regard as good parenting methods. We share with them our view that it can be misleading to describe parenting practices only in terms of "abusive" and "normal," because this assumes that abusive parents are somehow all the same, and that normal parents somehow are immune to the forces that create tension and anger between parents and children.

Parents are made aware of different "parenting styles" (discussed in Chapter 1)—a concept that generally carries less threatening connotations than "abuse" or "mistreatment." They are told that their child-rearing role involves, at a minimum, two very important functions: setting clear limits and establishing firm control for their children, and responding accurately and appropriately to their needs. Both functions are critical, because parents must control, direct, and stimulate their children, while attempting to understand and attend to each child's particular abilities and intentions. An example sometimes makes this clearer to clients:

> Suppose you woke up at night and heard your 2-year-old crying loudly. He doesn't usually do this, but you hate to be woken up. In this situation, which one of your "parent roles" would you draw upon: your role as the one who sets limits and maintains firm control, or your role as the one who responds to your child's needs of the moment? *(Parents typically identify their role as being the latter one in this situation.)*
>
> Now, let's say he does this screaming almost every night. You've had him to the pediatrician and there's nothing physically wrong with him. You've also checked on him many times, only to find that he's not suffering from any discomfort. He only seems to settle down if you stay in the room with him for 10–15 minutes. What role do you believe this calls for now? What would you do in such a situation?

At-risk parents tend to be "authoritarian" in their parenting style, in which they exhibit an insensitivity to their children's level of ability, interest, or needs, which can impair the children's developing self-esteem or motivation. In addition, at-risk or abusive parents may rely heavily on power-assertive techniques that overlook the children's current ability or readiness to learn (Oldershaw et al., 1986; Wolfe, 1987). To counter this tendency, parents are given the clear message that desirable child behavior does not occur by chance or solely because of a child's innate characteristics. Rather, parental *sensitivity* to the child's ongoing activity and readiness to comply will serve as an important factor influencing the child's willingness to cooperate. *Ipso facto*, firm control and preparedness are necessary qualities to ensure that rules and guidance have their intended effect.

Ineffective or inexperienced parents often benefit from establishing a clear "plan" in their minds, and rehearsing this plan many times until it becomes as automatic as their previous anger and arousal were. Consequently, we help them to develop a response to disciplinary situations that is adaptable to a variety of circumstances, and that anticipates (at least to some extent) the challenges that will emerge. Of course, no one "plan" fits all parents. Generally, we follow a simple outline based on the principle that parents will only use something if it is in line with their own thinking, makes intuitive sense, and provides additional direction.

To avoid the trap of having this strategy become only an "intellectual exercise," we teach it in an interactive fashion that presents familiar situations in an open-ended format. First, the therapist presents to parents a hierarchy of typical problem situations that require parental disciplinary action, beginning with minor infractions. Parents are asked to give their opinion as to what they would do and how effective their actions might be. The exercise is then reversed, and parents are given a chance to provide the situations while the therapist offers a suggested response. Following each extended "episode," therapist and parents view the videotape and discuss their choices, their intended effect, possible side effects, and possible "backup" alternatives.

Critical to this exercise is the fact that parents provide *their own preferred reaction*, no matter how inappropriate initially. Parents (and, alternatively, the therapist) are encouraged to defend their choices, their reasoning, and their attitudes against skepticism and challenge. In this manner the exercise can serve to bypass a common therapeutic dilemma, in which parents take on the role of skeptics and complainants, while the therapist attempts to dodge or attack every problem that is delivered.

The following example illustrates how a therapist may present increasingly challenging circumstances to a parent, in an attempt to elicit effective coping and problem resolution from him:

> John, before we begin this exercise, we should establish some principles for deciding how you will probably respond to something your child does. This will become your "plan," which will be refined and rehearsed many times in the clinic, and of course for years to come at home. First, we have to decide our

"threshold" for deciding that we should give the child a warning, follow through on punishment, and so on. How good are you at ignoring something your child does that is annoying or attention-seeking? It's better to act sooner than later, so let's establish right now what our rule should be for ignoring or not responding in any fashion to Billy's attention-seeking behavior *(Therapist discusses notion of children's acting out to get adult attention, and ways to redirect this behavior more constructively.)*

OK, now that we've more or less established *when* we should initiate a disciplinary action, let's establish our principles for this job. The first step is to determine for yourself what your mildest and your most powerful disciplinary actions should be, and then fill in the range of steps you can take in between these too end points. This range will determine your choices for *any and all child disciplinary actions* that you will take in the foreseen future. It is critical that you do not exceed this range once it is established, because doing so will uproot your entire plan and leave you much worse off than before. So think this over carefully, and let's write all your choices down. *(Therapist writes down the parent's preferred hierarchy and helps him to clarify his terms and options.)*

Next, you must figure out a strategy to help you decide, in each and every new situation, if the behavior in question warrants a disciplinary action, be it minor or major. Kids of all ages do things that can be bothersome, yet sometimes what they do is governed predominantly by their level of development. It might anger you considerably if your 3-year-old threw food at the table, but you have to expect such things from time to time from a 16-month-old. How are you going to decide if the behavior is within a "normal range" or acceptable limits, and what type of response it merits? This decision, of course, is often made so quickly it is almost reflexive, yet it still is *your choice and responsibility* to respond. To guide your actions, try to keep two simple questions in mind each and every time your child does something undesirable: "Can I reasonably expect this behavior to change?" If so, then remind yourself: "What's the best way to deal with this so that I don't get too upset?" If you're unsure of the answers, wait and talk it over with someone before responding!

To infuse some humor and realism into the exercise, parents are often reminded that children's "full-time occupation" is to seek out ways of exploring new frontiers, testing old rules, having a good time, and going about their business as they please. Parents may be just "blips" on their radar screen, so parents have to keep their presence known and look for ways to control and prevent the escalation of misbehavior early on. This "tracking" pays off handsomely as children mature.

All right, now let's put this into practice with some common situations involving children. All I want you to do is decide what, if any, response you would make to each situation. Because one form of punishment (or reward) is not enough for every situation, I urge you to use your full range of options as needed. I may ask for further details of exactly *how* you would do what you plan to do, or what changes you might make, especially if I add further complications (like, for example, if Billy doesn't go along with the program).

Let's begin with the problem you mentioned: Billy goes over and turns the TV set off and on. What response would you make to this now? (*Therapist makes every attempt to keep parent focused on his role, rather than "solving" the problem for him or just giving advice. The therapist's role is to encourage active problem solving, and to avoid "one-shot solutions" that fail to teach the disciplinary strategy adequately. Modeling or role playing may be substituted as needed. After parent offers response:*)

OK, you've told Billy firmly to stop turning off the TV set. He doesn't even notice you—he continues with this "game." Now what? (*Preferably, parent suggests a warning, with a consequence; if not, therapist continues to*

play out the situation anyway and leaves discussion until the
videotape review.) Once you've removed Billy from the
set, he goes over and hits his younger sister with a toy,
and she starts to scream. How are you feeling at this
point? Which option are you most likely to use now?
(Parent advises that he would be very angry, and would want
to use his "strongest hand"—putting Billy in the corner for
30 seconds.) It's not working to calm him down: Billy
screams louder and starts to kick at you and call you
names, saying he "hates you" over and over again. How
do you cope with this?

The therapist continues to challenge the parent's solutions in this
friendly scenario, designed to simulate a real-life episode.
However, because these circumstances do not elicit the emotional
reactions that would emerge in a real incident, the therapist is
primarily looking for the parent's ability to rely on the chosen
principles and strategy in the face of mounting defeat or
frustration. Parents are given the opportunity to rehearse more
true-to-life situations, complete with competing emotional
arousal, during subsequent exercises involving their own child
(see below). Finally, "turn about is fair play," so parents are given
an opportunity to reverse roles and experience the benign pleasure
of outfoxing and frustrating the therapist's intentions.

Anger Control and Rehearsal of
Disciplinary Encounters

Needless to say, it is important that parents be able to manage
their own anger and arousal before they attempt to modify their
discipline methods. Parents discuss with the therapist their
feelings of discomfort, tension, and frustration during disciplinary situations; their degree of motivation for learning how to
relax and handle situations more calmly is assessed. In our
experience, most parents are quite eager to learn how to relax, but
may be cautious about any technique that resembles "psychotherapy," "hypnosis," or "mind reading."

The process of anger control and discipline training begins

with parents' keeping a record of anger and arousal cues that occur at home over the week (in lieu of such a diary, we review the past week's events with them). We develop from this information an "anger profile," which includes antecedents to their anger, the setting that the anger often occurs in, the degree and type of response they show, and any consequences for such reactions (both good and bad consequences as perceived by the parents). Parents are then asked to attend a few sessions without the child present, in order to discuss their anger pattern and motivation for change. We determine what forms of relaxation or diversion they have attempted to use in the past, and how successful these methods are. We also determine whether parents are aware that their anger and arousal is escalating slowly, or whether they "suddenly lose their temper" and are insensitive to many of the earlier signs.

To begin the process of learning alternatives to physical punishment or angry threats, parents are asked to pick a recent situation involving their child that has led to considerable anger and upset on their part. They are then taught simple and brief relaxation skills, in an attempt to provide them with an alternative to arousal in the presence of this stressful situation (many parents enjoy this "break" once they have been introduced to it). The degree of relaxation achieved is often left to the control of the individual client, who provides feedback as to his or her comfort and enjoyment by verbal description and physical "cues" (some examples are provided in Koverola, Elliot-Faust, & Wolfe, 1984). We find that it is not necessary for a parent to use a particular relaxation procedure; rather, the parent should choose the approach that he or she is most comfortable with (e.g., visualization of pleasant scenes, deep muscle relaxation, breathing exercises).

Using a modified desensitization procedure, we introduce very gradually the stress-producing cues that the parents have identified, while they maintain a relaxed state. After reporting their ability to relax, they are encouraged to develop their individual strategy for self-control. We assist them in identifying self-statements that lead to greater self-control (e.g., "I know I can get through this if I just relax," "It ain't no big deal!"), and parents are asked to imagine ways of coping with the situation successfully. These exercises are repeated until a parent reports little arousal and believes that he or she has a way to cope with the imagined situation.

Typically, parents are now introduced to the use of nonphysical, noncoercive punishment procedures appropriate for the age and developmental level of their child. We review with parents individually the different methods of discipline that they have tried or are familiar with, and come to some agreement as to the methods they are most comfortable with. Parents often feel that they have tried just about everything with little success, but in fact they may have been inconsistent or inappropriate in how they implemented any changes (e.g., "I've tried putting him in his room—he just destroys things and makes such a fuss I have to let him out before I blow my top"). Although they may not have given some other methods a fair trial, their attitude toward any of these alternatives must be noted prior to suggesting their use. *Only methods that a parent has some degree of confidence in should be chosen for further instruction and application.*

We make no attempt to expose parents to the complete range of different punishment techniques and discipline strategies; rather, our goal is to assist them in developing their own comfortable style of reacting to difficult child behavior by using appropriate consequences and managing their arousal. If we overstructure the way in which punishment techniques are chosen and taught to parents, we run the risk of adding to their frustration and previous failures. We keep the verbal instructions to a minimum as well (typically, parents respond most favorably to rehearsing or observing real situations, and prefer not to read about, listen to, or discuss punishment methods for very long).

In terms of instruction per se, the basic "rules" of punishment are explained in simplest language:

- Punishment should be administered as soon as possible, usually immediately after the misbehavior.
- Punishment should involve natural consequences if at all possible (e.g., cleaning up one's own mess).
- Punishment should be preceded by a clear warning in most cases.
- Punishment should be at a level of intensity that fits the infraction.

We discuss with the parents at length how they might implement such an approach with their own child. Using their own examples, the parents are asked to describe how they can follow through on a recent conflict situation by using the punishment method they have chosen. Depending on the needs of each parent, individual training in relaxation and anger rehearsal may last from one to several sessions before they are introduced to live rehearsal in the presence of the child.

The rehearsal of punishment techniques poses a challenge to any parent training program, because we do not want a child to be frightened, unhappy, or unduly placed under duress. However, it is essential that parents have an opportunity to view the therapist modeling appropriate discipline with their child, and to rehearse their own style of discipline for future feedback and modification. In practice, there is no shortage of situations in which the child misbehaves to the point where some form of discipline is required. To rehearse such skills, a therapist often will request a child to terminate what he or she is doing and to focus on some less desirable task. With parents observing from behind the one-way mirror, the therapist then models appropriate discipline. The therapist avoids unnecessary criticism and provides acceptable alternatives to the child. Natural consequences are emphasized, which are extended to include loss of future privileges, cleaning up objects spilled, or removal from the play area if the child is disruptive.

For example, the therapist may state, "Bobby, you can either go back and finish what we asked you to do, or you can go and clean up the toys." Or the therapist may reinforce incompatible behavior in an attempt to defuse a problem situation (e.g., if the child is off task, the therapist may choose to distract the child to another activity and reinforce the child's attention to this activity). The therapist will also need to follow through with a predetermined consequence for noncompliance. Typically, this involves clearly stating to the child that what he or she is doing will not be allowed, and stating what will happen if the child does not comply. For a younger child, we commonly remove the child from the activity briefly by asking (or taking) him or her to sit on the couch for 10 or 15 seconds. If the situation deteriorates, we prefer for parents (and therapists) to "back off" gracefully, rather than attempting to increase the negative consequences. Only after parents have become very adept at following through in this manner will we introduce them to more restrictive forms of "time out" or removal from positive activities. This choice is based on our experience that such removal can become too coercive and physical, because a child will often kick and scream. Because of their anger control problems and/or lack of familiarity with young children, at-risk parents do best to err on the side of leniency, until such time as they can implement such consequences with minimal arousal and escalation.

Live rehearsal involving parents and their children alone together is a critical component of anger management. Parents need to rehearse their plans during "battle conditions," in order to gain confidence in being able to withstand the irritation and pressure that will occur from time to time with their child. The process is simple enough: The parents are brought back into the clinic playroom with their child; after some play activity, they make a request of the child that resembles common anger-eliciting situations (e.g., if they have problems getting the child to sit still and complete a task, we have them choose such an activity and demand that the child stay with the task in the clinic). Alternatively, the parents simply repeat a similar situation that was used with the therapist, in order for the therapist to determine how the parents follow through when noncompliance occurs. Further episodes are not provoked; rather, this rehearsal continues at home and during future clinic sessions spontaneously as common problems erupt.

Clinical Illustration

A clinical example can clarify some of these procedures. A 25-year-old single mother came to the clinic with a 4-year-old boy, who behaved very well when the mother was attending to him closely, but who would become quite noncompliant and destructive whenever the mother was engaged in another activity. Prior to discipline training, the mother had responded to his noncompliance in the clinic by repeating her commands over and over again, at which time the child would escalate his behavior and often start to hit the mother, in an attempt to get her to let him have his way. Some of these episodes would last as long as 10 minutes, at which time the therapist had to intervene to allow both parties to calm down.

The parent was taught brief relaxation training and a coping style, which involved self-statements of encouragement and guidance ("I know I can get through this," "I'm going to repeat this only once, and then follow through on what I've stated"). The parent chose to use a form of time out for the child, in which he was told to go and sit on the couch briefly. The mother would pick up a desirable toy and state to the child that as soon as he calmed down he could rejoin her on the floor and play with this toy.

This strategy worked very well for the parent: When the child began to misbehave, she made a clear request for compliance and followed this request up with a consequence if compliance was not forthcoming. Although the child began to throw temper tantrums while placed on the couch, he quickly regained his composure when the mother gave him an opportunity to rejoin the activity. Thus, after four sessions this problematic behavior occured only on occasion, and never for a very long time.

Treatment Termination: Winding Down and Following Through

Family problems that can lead to physical and emotional abuse are never fully "resolved" in the sense that they disappear and will never resurface. Risk of maltreatment is a fluid phenomenon that may wax and wane according to situational and individual factors, rather than a static factor that can be removed permanently. Therefore, the best strategy for terminating treatment is not to stop at all, but rather to maintain some level of involvement with the family on an ongoing basis. This professional commitment is nothing new in either mental health or physical health service delivery, and therefore is often perceived by parents as a more natural process of completion than establishing a final session. Furthermore, many of the skills and methods that have been taught require time to implement and evaluate; this allows for additional assistance at critical points in the future.

Deciding when a family's participation in treatment has come to a successful conclusion is based on a number of variables. This program does not establish an end point based on number of sessions, weeks elapsed, or particular skills demonstrated, because these fall short of covering the complexity of factors that go into such a decision. Like most forms of treatment, a decision to terminate is reached by mutual agreement between the primary therapist and the client(s). What complicates matters in this case, however, is the fact that such a decision often rests on the opinion of others outside of this therapist–client relationship. Therefore, the first consideration in deciding termination must be the terms of the original treatment agreement or contract (as discussed in Chapter 3). If the parents have followed through on the terms of this agreement, then the final decision to terminate treatment typically rests with the therapist and family directly. This responsibility is preferred, because the objectives set forth by the therapist typically involve less coercion and more family-directed assistance than those mandated by courts or child protection agencies, thus favoring a cooperative and issue-focused plan to wind down involvement.

Families complete treatment, therefore, on a gradual basis, beginning with the completion of the objectives noted in this and the preceding chapter. We realize that the training components of the program, which are often completed in anywhere from 12 weeks to a year, cannot provide adequate coverage of all the new or unresolved issues that face many high-risk families. Once a therapeutic relationship has become established over this period, however, the opportunities for long-term benefit are immense. In practical terms, a "fading out" of treatment, or a "follow-up visit" approach, is both sensible and realistic for evaluating the success of the treatment and offering ongoing services on an as-needed basis.

Maintaining contact with families requires mutual effort on the part of the therapist and parents. We begin by scheduling the last few appointments during the training phase at biweekly intervals, to permit time for generalization and to evaluate the lasting effects of observed changes more gradually. Therapists are encouraged to visit families in their homes more often at this point, for the purpose of observing the implementation of new skills as well as for purposes of outreach and commitment. Parents are encouraged to bring up enduring or newly encountered problems during each visit, and to take more and more of an active role in describing how they think they might resolve such problems. The therapist accordingly takes on a less direct and more supportive role, and seeks to direct parents to community resources that they can approach for the additional services they may require (e.g., day care, housing assistance, etc.). In many instances, this expanded role can be integrated with the role of the child protection agency social worker, who may be encouraged to keep the case "open" for the purpose of voluntary assistance rather than involuntary supervision.

In short, therapeutic contact should be faded out according to the needs and expectations of each family. Because each family differs in terms of what the parents had hoped to achieve or expected to see as a result of their participation, the extension of services should be made available in accordance with the family's interest and consent in maintaining ongoing contact. Not only is the risk of abuse substantially decreased through such contact (by nature of the process of monitoring family developments), but this also affords parents greater opportunities to rehearse new skills and establish more healthy styles of interaction.

Looking Ahead

The evolution of child abuse prevention and treatment methods is far from complete. We are just beginning to develop strategies that move beyond the narrow realm of treating the parents' inappropriate attitudes and behaviors, to take into account the needs of the child (Kaufman & Rudy, 1991; Rosenberg & Reppucci, 1985) and the importance of addressing the family's limited resources and supports (Garbarino, 1987). Long-standing forms of intervention that disrupt or impair the ongoing parent–child relationship (e.g., removal of the child from the home), which can create a worse situation in some respects, have been called into question by some researchers (e.g., Melton, 1990;

Wald, Carlsmith, & Liederman, 1988). There is general agreement that no single strategy can be expected to work with the diversity of families and circumstances encountered with this population. Therefore, it is critical that practitioners, community planners, and government agencies carefully consider recent developments that offer considerable insights for formulating promising intervention and prevention programs.

The program described in this volume is grounded in the belief that the goal of preventing child abuse can be best achieved by maximizing children's developmental abilities through child-centered stimulation activities involving the parents. This strategy is based on research findings with abused children, which indicate that the effects of abuse are cumulative over time, creating something of a domino effect on subsequent development (Aber & Cicchetti, 1984; Shirk, 1988). Without early intervention, a child's development may be delayed or disrupted by the everyday actions taken by a parent who is not sensitive to the child's needs and abilities. Thus, isolated episodes of violence or rejection may be only the *visible markers* of a disturbed parent–child relationship. For intervention purposes, we must look beyond these events to consider the overall parent–child relationship and ways in which it can be improved for the sake of healthy child development.

The developmental orientation underlying our intervention program implies something of a departure from most current efforts to treat child victims of maltreatment and to prevent its recurrence. First of all, practitioners can consider a child's symptoms as reflecting his or her efforts to learn social behaviors without the benefit of sensitive parenting or careful guidance, and thereby can direct intervention more toward the strengthening of developmentally relevant tasks or skills, in addition to specific presenting complaints. Equally important is the implication, based on this orientation, that prevention and intervention efforts can be planned from an earlier point in time in such a way that undersirable (and potentially problematic) developmental deficits can be minimized. Rather than relying on aversive contingencies (i.e., detecting abuse and neglect and imposing changes on the family), a developmentally guided intervention/prevention strategy works on the principle of providing the least intrusive, earliest assistance possible. The focus is shifted away from identifying misdeeds of a parent, and more toward promoting an optimal balance between the needs of a child and the abilities and resources of a family.

Research and practice over the past two decades have considerably advanced our understanding and awareness of physical and emotional abuse of children. With this expanding knowledge base, major goals of prevention-focused direct-service programs have been clarified (e.g., increasing parents' knowledge of child development and the demands of parenting; enhancing parents' skill in coping with stress related to caring for small children; enhancing parent–child attachment and communication; increasing parents' knowledge of home management; reducing/sharing the burden of child care; and increasing access to social and health services for all family members; Wolfe, in press). With these goals in mind, what are some key social policy factors in the long-term success of direct-service child abuse prevention programs?

One key factor in the success of prevention programs is the recognition of the need of all families for support and education. Adequate supports, both instrumental and emotional, are important for the healthy functioning of families. Such supportive services should include, at a minimum, formal, agency-based services; quasi-formal supports (e.g., self-help groups); and informal supports that are accessible to individual families. The challenge remains to expand existing family support servcices, with their range of concrete, social, and psychological services, to more "at-risk" families who have poor histories of child care and a poor record of meeting responsibilities successfully (e.g., employment). The advantage of a family support (i.e., enhancement) strategy, in contrast to an interception approach, is that it provides a blend of services in a family-centered format. Such a model, however, requires different allocations of resources and professional commitment than the ones presently in place (Wolfe, 1990).

A second key factor influencing the future success of prevention programs is the clarification of our community values and our prevention orientation. Better-defined guidelines are needed for establishing what the minimum standards of care should be, and when official intervention is seen as a necessary step. Similarly, the willingness of different communities to implement family support programs at a broader and more comprehensive level must be addressed. Such programs are aimed at preventing the breakdown of families that require alternative care, and evidence is emerging as to their efficacy and impact on positive child and family development (e.g., Olds, Henderson, Chamberlain, & Tatelbaum, 1986; Wald et al., 1988). Social scientists emphasize that social support systems are the mechanisms by which corrective measures for families are naturally provided; yet such systems may require our deliberate planning and implementation, to ensure that families receive adequate nurturance and feedback on their child rearing.

Most forms of family violence toward children (i.e., physical abuse, exposure to wife assault, and psychological abuse), as well as child-rearing inadequacies (e.g., emotional and physical neglect), entail many of the actions and circumstances that are indicative of socialization failure. Therefore, a critical need exists to discover and implement different ways of preventing such failure well in advance of the establishment of abusive and rejecting patterns of childrearing. This prevention task is now a distinct possibility, in view of our acquired knowledge of the social and psychological causes of maltreatment; thus, a top priority should be to formulate, implement, and evaluate the effectiveness of prevention-oriented family support programs. Such a strategy is a recognized move away from our existing approach: Rather than continuing to work within a system that necessitates a serious breach in legally acceptable child care before intervention is applied, we should be making responsive and proactive efforts toward family development and acknowledgment of unique cultural distinctions. We have entered a time in which there is a re-emphasis on family integrity, as opposed to out-of-home placements, and in conjunction with this movement social service and mental health agencies are looking for ways to offer assistance to families (whether intact, single-parent, or reconstituted) that will eliminate or reduce the need for protective supervision.

Finally, we should encourage diversity of styles and opportunities for the development of unique resources for children and parents. High-risk parents are extremely diverse in their needs, and not all will "fit" into a training program or welcome family assistance in child rearing. These issues will require a new model or paradigm to approach the complexity of parental needs, since the view that all child abusers are alike has not been supported. Prevention efforts should not be limited to identified "high-risk" populations or those who are currently faced with child-rearing responsibilities; we must encourage more awareness of family life roles and responsibilities during adolescence and young adulthood, and strive to involve males more often in educational efforts. Such objectives may be achieved by developing interesting materials and opportunities to engage young adults early in the formation of their attitudes and behaviors toward family members.

References

Aber, J. L., & Allen, J. P. (1987). Effects of maltreatment on young children's socioemotional development: An attachment theory perspective. *Developmental Psychology, 23*, 406–414.

Aber, J. L., & Cicchetti, D. (1984). The socio-emotional development of maltreated children: An empirical and theoretical analysis. In H. Fitzgerald, B. Lester, & M. Yogman (Eds.), *Theory and research in behavioral pediatrics* (Vol. 2, pp. 147–205). New York: Plenum.

Abidin, R. (1983). *The Parenting Stress Index.* Charlottesville, VA: Pediatric Psychology Press.

Achenbach, T., & Edelbrock, C. S. (1983). *Manual for the Child Behavior Checklist and Revised Child Behavior Profile.* Burlington: University of Vermont, Department of Psychiatry.

Ainsworth, M., Blehar, M., Waters, E., & Wall, S. (1978). *Patterns of attachment: A psychological study of the strange situation.* Hillsdale, NJ: Erlbaum.

Ambrose, S., Hazzard, A., & Haworth, J. (1980). Cognitive–behavioral parenting groups for abusive families. *Child Abuse & Neglect, 4,* 119–125.

American Humane Association (AHA). (1984). *Trends in child abuse and neglect: A national perspective.* Denver, CO: Author.

Ammerman, R.T. (1990). Etiological models of child maltreatment: A behavioral perspective. *Behavior Modification, 14,* 230–254.

Ammerman, R.T. (in press). The role of the child in physical abuse: A reappraisal. *Violence and Victims.*

Anisfeld, E., Casper, V., Nozyce, M., & Cunningham, N. (1990). Does infant carrying promote attachment? An experimental study of the effects of increased physical contact on the development of attachment. *Child Development, 61,* 1617–1627.

Appelbaum, A.S. (1977). Developmental retardation in infants as a concomitant of physical child abuse. *Journal of Abnormal Child Psychology, 5*, 417–423.

Aronson, H., & Overall, B. (1966). Treatment expectations of parents in two social classes. *Social Work, 11*, 35–41.

Averill, J.R. (1983). Studies on anger and aggression: Implications for theories of emotion. *American Psychologist, 38*, 1145–1160.

Azar, S. T. (1989). Training parents of abused children. In C.E. Schaefer & J.M. Briesmeister (Eds.), *Handbook of parent training: Parents as co-therapists for children's behavior problems* (pp. 414–441). New York: Wiley.

Azar, S. T., Robinson, D.R., Hekimian, E., & Twentyman, C.T. (1984). Unrealistic expectations and problem-solving ability in maltreating and comparison mothers. *Journal of Consulting and Clinical Psychology, 52*, 687–691.

Azar, S. T., & Rohrbeck, C. A. (1986). Child abuse and unrealistic expectations: Further validation of the Parent Opinion Questionnaire. *Journal of Consulting and Clinical Psychology, 54*, 867–868.

Azar, S.T., & Siegel, B.R. (1990). Behavioral treatment of child abuse: A developmental perspective. *Behavior Modification, 14*, 279–300.

Azar, S.T., & Wolfe, D.A. (1989). Child abuse and neglect. In E.J. Mash & R.A. Barkley (Eds.), *Behavioral treatment of childhood disorders* (pp. 451–489). New York: Guilford Press.

Barkley, R. A. (1987). *Defiant children: A clinician's manual for parent training.* New York: Guilford Press.

Bauer, W. D., & Twentyman, C. T. (1985). Abusing, neglectful, and comparison mothers' responses to child-related and non-child-related stressors. *Journal of Consulting and Clinical Psychology, 53*, 335–343.

Baumrind, D. (1971). Current patterns of parental authority. *Developmental Psychology Monographs, 4*(1, Pt. 2).

Bell, G. (1973). Parents who abuse their children. *Canadian Psychiatric Association Journal, 18*, 223–228.

Bell, R. Q., & Harper, L. (1977). *Child effects on adults.* Hillsdale, NJ: Erlbaum.

Belsky, J. (1980). Child maltreatment: An ecological integration. *American Psychologist, 35*, 320–335.

Berkowitz, L. (1983). Aversively stimulated aggression: Some parallels and differences in research with animals and humans. *American Psychologist, 38*, 1135–1144.

Berkowitz, L. (1990). On the formation and regulation of anger and aggression: A cognitive–neoassociationistic analysis. *American Psy-*

chologist, 45, 494–503.

Besharov, D. J. (1985). *Child abuse and neglect law: A Canadian perspective.* Washington, DC: Child Welfare League of America.

Blumberg, M.L. (1974). Psychopathology of the abusing parent. *American Journal of Psychotherapy, 28,* 21–29.

Bornstein, M., & Tamis-LeMonda, C. (1989). Maternal responsiveness and cognitive development in children. In M. Bornstein (Ed.), New directions for child development: No. 43. *Maternal responsiveness: Characteristics and consequences.* San Francisco: Jossey-Bass. (pp. 49–61).

Bousha, D.M., & Twentyman, C.T. (1984). Mother–child interactional style in abuse, neglect, and control groups: Naturalistic observations in the home. *Journal of Abnormal Psychology, 93,* 106–114.

Brassard, M. R., Germain, R., & Hart, S. N. (Eds.). (1987). *Psychological maltreatment of children and youth.* New York: Pergamon.

Brewin, C. R. (1989). Cognitive change processes in psychotherapy. *Psychological Review, 96,* 379–394.

Brooks-Gunn, J., & Lewis, M. (1984). Maternal responsivity in interactions with handicapped infants. *Child Development, 55,* 782–793.

Burgess, R.L. (1979). Child abuse: A social interactional analysis. In B.B. Lahey & A. Kazdin (Eds.), *Advances in clinical child psychology* (Vol. 2, pp. 142–172). New York: Plenum.

Burgess, R.L., & Conger, R. (1978). Family interactions in abusive, neglectful, and normal families. *Child Development, 49,* 1163–1173.

Campbell, D. (1989). About discipline and punishment: An examination of corporal punishment and child development. In M. Clarke (Ed.), *Policies for children in the '90s: A Canadian series.* Ottawa: Canadian Council on Children and Youth. Child and Family Services Act, Ontario Revised Statutes (19).

Children's Aid Society (CAS) of the Region of Peel [Ontario]. (1988). *Position paper on physical discipline.* Unpublished manuscript.

Child and Family Services Act. (1984). *Statutes of Ontario,* Chapter 55. Toronto: Queen's Printer.

Cicchetti, D. (1989). How research on child maltreatment has informed the study of child development: Perspectives from developmental psychopathology. In D. Cicchetti & V. Carlson (Eds.), *Child maltreatment: Theory and research on the causes and consequences of child abuse and neglect* (pp. 377–431). New York: Cambridge University Press.

Cicchetti, D., & Rizley, R. (1981). Developmental perspectives on the etiology, intergenerational transmission, and sequelae of child maltreatment. In D. Cicchetti & R. Rizley (Eds.), *New directions for child development: Developmental perspectives on child maltreatment* (pp. 31–55). San Francisco: Jossey-Bass.

Cicchetti, D., Toth, S., & Bush, M. (1988). Developmental psychopathology and incompetence in childhood: Suggestions for intervention. In B.B. Lahey & A.E. Kazdin (Eds.), *Advances in clinical child psychology* (Vol. 11, pp. 1–77). New York: Plenum.

Clark, G.N., & Seifer, R. (1983). Facilitating mother–infant communication: A treatment model for high-risk and developmentally delayed infants. *Infant Mental Health Journal, 4*, 67–82.

Coates, D.L., & Lewis, M. (1984). Early mother–infant interaction and infant cognitive status as predictors of school performance and cognitive behavior in six year olds. *Child Development, 55*, 1219–1230.

Cohn, A.H. (1979). Essential elements of successful child abuse and neglect treatment. *Child Abuse & Neglect, 3*, 491–496.

Cone, J. D. (1984). *The Pyramid Scales: Criterion-referenced measures of adaptive behavior in handicapped persons.* Austin, TX: Pro-Ed.

Conger, R. D., Burgess, R., & Barrett, C. (1979). Child abuse related to life change and perceptions of illness: Some preliminary findings. *Family Coordinator, 28*, 73–78.

Corson, J., & Davidson, H. (1987). Emotional abuse and the law. In M. Brassard, R. Germain, & S. Hart (Eds.), *Psychological maltreatment of children and youth* (pp. 185–202). New York: Pergamon.

Covell, K., & Abramovitch, R. (1987). Understanding emotion in the family: Children's and parents' attributions of happiness, madness, and anger. *Child Development, 58*, 985–991.

Crittenden, P.M. (1988). Relationships at risk. In J. Belsky & T. Nezworski (Eds.), *Clinical implications of attachment theory* (pp. 136–174). Hillsdale, NJ: Erlbaum.

Crittenden, P.M., & Bonvillian, J.D. (1984). The relationship between maternal risk status and maternal sensitivity. *American Journal of Orthopsychiatry, 54*, 250–262.

Crittenden, P.M., & Snell, M. (1983). Intervention to improve mother–infant interaction and infant development. *Infant Mental Health Journal, 4*, 23–31.

Crnic, K., Greenberg, M., Ragozin, A., Robinson, N., & Basham, R. (1983). Effects of stress and social support on mothers and premature and full-term infants. *Child Development, 54*, 209–217.

Daro, D. (1990). *Confronting child abuse: Research for effective program design.* New York: Free Press.

Dietrich, K.N., Starr, R.H., & Kaplan, M.G. (1980). Maternal stimulation and care of abused infants. In T.M. Field, S. Goldberg, D. Stern, & A.M. Sostek (Eds.), *High-risk infants and children: Adult and peer interactions* (pp. 25–41). New York: Academic Press.

Denicola, J., & Sandler, J. (1980). Training abusive parents in cognitive–behavioral techniques. *Behavior Therapy, 11*, 263–270.

Disbrow, M.A., Doerr, H., & Caulfield, C. (1977). Measuring the components of parents' potential for child abuse and neglect. *Child Abuse & Neglect, 1*, 279–296.

Egan, K. (1983). Stress management and child management with abusive parents. *Journal of Clinical Child Psychology, 12*, 292–299.

Egeland, B., & Sroufe, A. (1981). Attachment and early maltreatment. *Child Development, 52*, 44–52.

Elmer, E. (1963). Identification of abused children. *Children, 10*, 180–184.

Emde, R. (1988). Development terminable and interminable: I. Innate and motivational factors from infancy. *International Journal of Psycho-Analysis, 68*, 3–22.

Erickson, M.F., Sroufe, L.A., & Egeland, B. (1985). The relationship between quality of attachment and relationship problems in preschool in a high-risk sample. *Monographs of the Society for Research in Child Development*, In I. Bretherton & E. Waters (Eds.), *50*(1–2), 147–166.

Fantuzzo, J. W. (1990). Behavioral treatment of the victims of child abuse and neglect. *Behavior Modification, 14*, 316–339.

Forehand, R.L., & McMahon, R.J. (1981). *Helping the noncompliant child: A clinician's guide to parent training*. New York: Guilford Press.

Foster, S. L., & Robin, A. L. (1988). Family conflict and communication in adolescents. In E. J. Mash & L. G. Terdal (Eds.), *Behavioral assessment of childhood disorders* (2nd ed., pp. 717–775). New York: Guilford Press.

Fraiberg, S. (1974). Blind infants and their mothers: An examination of sign system. In M. Lewis & L. Rosenblum (Eds.), *The effect of the infant on its caregiver* (pp. 215–232). New York: Wiley.

Frodi, A., & Lamb, M. (1980). Child abusers' responses to infant smiles and cries. *Child Development, 51*, 238–241.

Gaines, R., Sandgrund, A., Green, A. H., & Power, E. (1978). Etiological factors in child maltreatment: A multivariate study of abusing, neglecting, and normal mothers. *Journal of Abnormal Psychology, 87*, 531–541.

Garbarino, J. (1977). The human ecology of child maltreatment: A conceptual model for research. *Journal of Marriage and the Family, 39*, 721–735.

Garbarino, J. (1987). Family support and the prevention of child maltreatment. In S. L. Kagan, D. R. Powell, B. Weissbourd, & E. F. Zigler (Eds.), *America's family support programs* (pp. 99–114). New Haven, CT: Yale University Press.

Garbarino, J., Guttman, E., & Seeley, J. (1986). *The psychologically battered child.* San Francisco: Jossey-Bass.

Gelles, R. J. (1973). Child abuse as psychopathology: A sociological critique and reformulation. *American Journal of Orthopsychiatry, 43,* 611–621.

George, C., & Main, M. (1979). Social interactions of young abused children: Approach, avoidance, and aggression. *Child Development, 50,* 306–318.

Gil, D.G. (1970). *Violence against children: Physical child abuse in the United States.* Cambridge, MA: Harvard University Press.

Green, A.H. (1976). A psychdynamic approach to the study and treatment of child-abusing parents. *Journal of the Academy of Child Psychiatry, 15,* 414–429.

Green, A.H. (1978). Child abuse. In B.B. Wolman, J. Egan, & A. Ross (Eds.), *Handbook of treatment of mental disorders in childhood and adolescence* (pp. 430–455). Englewood Cliffs, NJ: Prentice-Hall.

Green, A.H., Gaines, R.W., & Sandgrund, A. (1974). Child abuse: Pathological syndrome of family interaction. *American Journal of Psychiatry, 131,* 882–886.

Hann, D., Osofsky, J., & Carter, S. (1990, April). *A comparison of effects between infants of adolescent and older mothers.* Paper presented at the International Conference on Infant Studies, Montreal.

Hansen, D. J., & MacMillan, V. M. (1990). Behavioral assessment of child-abusive and neglectful families. *Behavior Modification, 14,* 255–278.

Hanson, D. J., Pallotta, G. M., Tishelman, A. C., Conaway, L. P., & MacMillan, V. M. (1989). Parental problem-solving skills and child behavior problems: A comparison of physically abusive, neglectful, clinic, and community families. *Journal of Family Violence, 4,* 353–368.

Hart, S. N., Germain, R., & Brassard, M. R., (1987). The challenge: To better understand and combat psychological maltreatment of children and youth. In M. R. Brassard, R. Germain, & S. N. Hart (Eds.), *Psychological maltreatment of children and youth* (pp. 3–24). New York: Pergamon.

Helfer, R.E. (1973). The etiology of child abuse. *Pediatrics, 51,* 777.

Herrenkohl, R.C., Herrenkohl, E.C., & Egolf, B.P. (1983). Circumstances surrounding the occurrence of child maltreatment. *Journal of*

Consulting and Clinical Psychology, 51, 424–431.

Herrenkohl, R.C., Herrenkohl, E.C., Egolf, B.P., & Seech, M. (1979). The repetition of child abuse: How frequently does it occur? *Child Abuse & Neglect, 3*, 67–72.

Institute for the Prevention of Child Abuse. (1989, January). Survey of Canadian parental attitudes. *Newsbrief* (Available from 25 Spadina Road, Toronto, Ontario M5R 2S9).

Isaacs, C.D. (1982). Treatment of child abuse: A review of the behavioral interventions. *Journal of Applied Behavior Analysis, 15*, 273–294.

Jaffe, P., Wolfe, D. A., & Wilson, S. (1990). *Children of battered women*. Newbury Park, CA: Sage.

Jones, M.A. (1987). *A second chance for families: Five years later--Follow-up of a program to prevent foster care*. New York: Child Welfare League of America.

Kaufman, I. R. (1977). Standards relating to abuse and neglect. In I. R. Kaufman (Chair), *Institute of Judicial Administration--American Bar Association Joint Commission on Juvenile Justice Standards*. Cambridge, MA: Ballinger.

Kaufman, J., & Zigler, E. (1989). The intergenerational transmission of child abuse and the prospect of predicting future abusers. In D. Cicchetti & V. Carlson (Eds.), *Child maltreatment: Research and theory on the causes and consequences of child abuse and neglect* (pp. 129–150). New York: Cambridge University Press.

Kaufman, K. L., & Rudy, L. (1991). Future directions in the treatment of physical child abuse. *Criminal Justice and Behavior, 18*, 82–97.

Kaye, K. (1982). *The mental and social life of babies*. Chicago: University of Chicago Press.

Kazdin, A. E. (1988). *Child psychotherapy: Developing and identifying effective treatments*. New York: Pergamon Press.

Kelly, J.A. (1983). *Treating abusive families: Intervention based on skills training principles*. New York: Plenum.

Kempe, C.H., & Helfer, R.E. (1972). *Helping the battered child and his family*. Philadelphia: Lippincott.

Kempe, C.H., Silverman, F.N., Steele, B.F., Droegenmueller, W., & Silver, H.K. (1962). The battered child syndrome. *Journal of the American Medical Association, 181*, 17–24.

Koverola, C., Elliot-Faust, D., & Wolfe, D. A. (1984). Clinical issues in the behavioral treatment of a child abusive mother experiencing multiple life stresses. *Journal of Clinical Child Psychology, 13*, 187–191.

Krupka, A., & Moran, G. (1991). [The quality of mother–infant interactions in families at risk for maladaptive parenting: Maternal sensitivity as an avenue for primary prevention of child maltreatment]. Unpublished raw data, Department of Psychology, The University of Western Ontario.

Lahey, B.B., Conger, R.D., Atkeson, B.M., & Treiber, F.A. (1984). Parenting behavior and emotional status of physically abusive mothers. *Journal of Consulting and Clinical Psychology, 52,* 1062–1071.

Lamb, M., & Easterbrooks, M.A. (1981). Individual differences in parental sensitivity: Origins, components, and consequences. In M.E. Lamb & K.R. Sherrod (Eds.), *Infant social cognition: Theoretical and empirical considerations* (pp. 127–154). Hillsdale, NJ: Erlbaum.

LaRose, L., & Wolfe, D.A. (1987). Psychological characteristics of parents who abuse or neglect their children. In B.B. Lahey & A.E. Kazdin (Eds.), *Advances in clinical child psychology* (Vol. 10, pp. 55–97). New York: Plenum.

Larrance, D.T., & Twentyman, C.T. (1983). Maternal attributions and child abuse. *Journal of Abnormal Psychology, 92,* 449–457.

Lauer, J. W., Lourie, I. S., Salus, M. K., & Broadhurst, D. D. (1979). *The role of the mental health professional in the prevention and treatment of child abuse and neglect.* Washington, DC: Department of Health, Education and Welfare.

Lewis, M., & Coates, D.L. (1980). Mother–infant interaction and cognitive development in twelve-week-old infants. *Infant Behavior and Development, 3,* 95–105.

Light, R. (1973). Abused and neglected children in America: A study of alternative policies. *Harvard Educational Review, 43,* 556–598.

Lorber, R., Felton, D.K., & Reid, J. (1984). A social learning approach to the reduction of coercive processes in child abusive families: A molecular analysis. *Advances in Behaviour Research and Therapy, 6,* 29–45.

Loyd, B., & Abidin, R. (1985). Revision of the Parenting Stress Index. *Journal of Pediatric Psychology, 10,* 169–177.

Lutzker, J. R. (1984). Project 12-Ways: Treating child abuse and neglect from an ecobehavioral perspective. In R.F. Dangel & R.A. Polster (Eds.), *Parent training: Foundations of research and practice* (pp. 260–295). New York: Guilford Press.

Lutzker, J. R., & Rice, J. M. (1984). Project 12-Ways: Measuring outcome of a large in-home service for treatment and prevention of child abuse and neglect. *Child Abuse & Neglect, 8,* 519–524.

Maccoby, E.E., & Martin, J.A. (1983). Socialization in the context of the family: Parent–child interaction. In E.M. Hetherington (Ed.), *Handbook of child psychology* (4th ed.): *Vol. 4. Socialization, personality, and social development* (pp. 1–101). New York: Wiley.

Magnuson, E. (1983, September 5). Child abuse: The ultimate betrayal. *Time*, pp. 16–18.

Mahrer, A., Levinson, J., & Fine, S. (1976). Infant psychotherapy: Theory, research, and practice. *Psychotherapy: Theory, Research, and Practice, 13*, 131–140.

Main, M., Kaplan, R., & Cassidy, J. (1985). Security in infancy, childhood, and adulthood: A move to the level of representation. In I. Bretherton & E. Waters (Eds.), Growing points of attachment theory and research. *Monographs of the Society for Research in Child Development, 50* (1–2, Serial No. 209).

Mash, E.J., Johnston, C., & Kovitz, K. (1983). A comparison of the mother–child interactions of physically abused and non-abused children during play and task situations. *Journal of Clinical Child Psychology, 12*, 337–346.

Mash, E. J., & Wolfe, D. A. (1991). Methodological issues in research on physical child abuse. *Criminal Justice and Behavior, 18*, 8–30.

McGee, R., & Wolfe, D. A. (1991). Psychological maltreatment: Towards an operational definition. *Development and Psychopathology, 3*, 3–18.

Melnick, B., & Hurley, J.R. (1969). Distinctive personality attributes of child-abusing mothers. *Journal of Consulting and Clinical Psychology, 33*, 746–749.

Melton, G.B. (1990). Child protection: Making a bad situation worse? *Contemporary Psychology, 35*, 213–214.

Merrill, E. J. (1962). Physical abuse of children: An agency study. In V. DeFrancis (Ed.), *Protecting the battered child*. Denver, CO: American Humane Association.

Miller, S.A. (1988). Parents' beliefs about children's cognitive development. *Child Development, 59*, 259–285.

Milner, J. S. (1986). *The Child Abuse Potential Inventory: Manual*. Webster, NC: Psytec.

Milner, J. S. (1991). Physical child abuse perpetrator screening and evaluation. *Criminal Justice and Behavior, 18*, 47–63.

Milner, J.S., & Wimberley, R.C. (1980). Prediction and explanation of child abuse. *Journal of Clinical Psychology, 36*, 875–884.

Morris, M., & Gould, R. (1963). Role reversal: A necessary concept in dealing with the battered child syndrome. *American Journal of Orthopsychiatry, 33*, 298–299.

National Center on Child Abuse and Neglect (NCCAN). (1981). *Study findings: National study of the incidence and severity of child abuse and neglect*. Washington, DC: U.S. Government Printing Office.

National Center on Child Abuse and Neglect (NCCAN). (1988). *Study findings: Study of the national incidence of and prevalence of child abuse and neglect*. Washington, DC: U.S. Government Printing Office.

Oldershaw, L., Walters, G. C., & Hall, D. K. (1986). Control strategies and noncompliance in abusive mother–child dyads: An observational study. *Child Development, 57,* 722–732.

Olds, D.L., & Henderson, C.R. (1989). The prevention of maltreatment. In D. Cicchetti & V. Carlson (Eds.), *Child maltreatment: Theory and research on the causes and consequences of child abuse and neglect* (pp. 722–763). NY: Cambridge University Press.

Olds, D.L., Henderson, C.R., Chamberlain, R., & Tatelbaum, R. (1986). Preventing child abuse and neglect. *Pediatrics, 78,* 65–78.

Parke, R.D. (1977). Socialization into child abuse: A social interactional perspective. In J.L. Tapp & F.J. Levine (Eds.), Law, justice, and the individual in society: Psychological and legal issues (pp. 183–199). New York: Holt, Rinehart & Winston.

Parke, R.D., & Collmer, C.W. (1975). Child abuse: An interdisciplinary analysis. In E.M. Hetherington (Ed.), *Review of child development research* (Vol. 5, pp. 509–590). Chicago: University of Chicago Press.

Patterson, G.R. (1982). *Coercive family process*. Eugene, OR: Castalia.

Patterson, G.R., Reid, J.B., Jones, R.R., & Conger, R.E. (1975). *A social learning approach to family intervention*: Vol. 1. *Families with aggressive children*. Champaign, IL: Research Press.

Pelton, L.H. (1978). Child abuse and neglect: The myth of classlessness. *American Journal of Orthopsychiatry, 48,* 608–617.

Pennebaker, J. W. (1985). Traumatic experience and psychosomatic disease: Exploring the roles of behavioral inhibition, obsession, and confiding. *Canadian Psychology, 26,* 82–95.

Radbill, S.X. (1968). A history of child abuse and infanticide. In R.E. Helfer & C.H. Kempe (Eds.), *The battered child* (pp. 3–17). Chicago: University of Chicago Press.

Reid, J.B., Taplin, P., & Lorber, R. (1981). A social interactional approach to the treatment of abusive families. In R.B. Stuart (Ed.), *Violent behavior: Social learning approaches to prediction, management, and treatment* (pp. 83–101). New York: Brunner/Mazel.

Rosenberg, M.S. (1987). New directions for research on the psychological maltreatment of children. *American Psychologist, 42,* 166–171.

Rosenberg, M.S., & Reppucci, N.D. (1985). Primary prevention of child abuse. *Journal of Consulting and Clinical Psychology, 53,* 576–585.

Salzinger, S., Kaplan, S., & Artemyeff, C. (1983). Mothers' personal social networks and child maltreatment. *Journal of Abnormal Psychology, 92,*

68–76.

Sameroff, A., & Chandler, M. (1975). Reproductive risk and the continuum of caretaking casualty. In F. Horowitz (Ed.), *Review of child development research* (Vol. 4, pp. 197–244). Chicago: University of Chicago Press.

Sattler, J. M. (1988). *Assessment of children* (3rd ed.). San Diego, CA: Author.

Shaw-Lamphear, V.S. (1985). The impact of maltreatment on children's psychosocial adjustment: A review of the research. *Child Abuse & Neglect, 9*, 251–263.

Shirk, S. R. (1988). The interpersonal legacy of physical abuse of children. In M. Straus (Ed.), *Abuse and victimization across the lifespan.* (pp. 57–81). Baltimore: Johns Hopkins University Press.

Smith, P., & Pederson, D. (1988). Maternal sensitivity and patterns of infant–mother attachment. *Child Development, 56*, 1–14.

Spinetta, J.J. (1978). Parental personality factors in child abuse. *Journal of Consulting and Clinical Psychology, 46*, 1409–1414.

Spinetta, J.J., & Rigler, D. (1972). The child abusing parent: A psychological review. *Psychological Bulletin, 77*, 296–304.

Sroufe, L.A., & Fleeson, J. (1986). Attachment and the construction of relationships. In W.W. Hartup & Z. Rubin (Eds.), *Relationships and development* (pp. 51–71). Hillsfale, NJ: Erlbaum.

Starr, R.H., Jr. (1979). Child abuse. *American Psychologist, 34*, 872–878.

Starr, R.H., Jr. (1982). A research-based approach to the prediction of child abuse. In R.H. Starr, Jr. (Ed.), *Child abuse prediction: Policy implications* (pp. 105–134). Cambridge, MA: Ballinger.

Steele, B. J., & Pollock, C. (1968). A psychiatric study of parents who abuse infants and small children. In R. Helfer & C.H. Kempe (Eds.), *The battered child* (pp. 89–133). Chicago: University of Chicago Press.

Stern, D. N. (1977). *The first relationship.* Cambridge, England: Cambridge University Press.

Stevens, J. H. (1984). Black grandmothers' and black adolescent mothers' knowledge about parenting. *Developmental Psychology, 20*, 1017–1025.

Straus, M.A., Gelles, R.J., & Steinmetz, S. (1980). *Behind closed doors: Violence in the American family.* Garden City, NY: Doubleday/Anchor.

Susman, E.J., Trickett, P.K., Iannotti, R.J., Hollenbeck, B.E., & Zahn-Waxler, C. (1985). Child-rearing patterns in depressed, abusive, and normal mothers. *American Journal of Orthopsychiatry, 55*, 237–251.

Szykula, S. A., & Fleischman, M. J. (1985). Reducing out-of-home placement for abused children: Two controlled studies. *Child Abuse & Neglect, 9*, 277–284.

Trickett, P. K., & Kuczynski, L. (1986). Children's misbehaviors and parental discipline strategies in abusive and nonabusive families. *Developmental Psychology, 22,* 115–123.

Wald, M.S., Carlsmith, J.M., & Liederman, P.H. (1988). *Protecting abused and neglected children.* Stanford, CA: Stanford University Press.

Wasserman, S. (1967). The abused parent of the abused child. *Children, 14,* 175–179.

Watson, D., & Pennebaker, J. W. (1989). Health complaints, stress, and distress: Exploring the central role of negative affectivity. *Psychological Review, 96,* 234–254.

Watson, J. (1979). Perception of contingency as a determinant of social responsiveness. In E. B. Thomas (Ed.), *Origins of the infant's social responsiveness* (pp. 33–64). Hillsdale, NJ: Erlbaum.

Watson, J. (1985). Contingency perception in early social development. In T. Field & N. N. Fox (Eds.), *Social perceptions in children* (pp. 157–176). Norwood, NJ: Ablex.

Wedell-Monnig, J., & Lumley, J. M. (1980). Child deafness and mother–child interaction. *Child Development, 51,* 766–774.

Wekerle, C., & Wolfe, D.A. (1991). *An empirical review of prevention strategies for child abuse and neglect.* Manuscript submitted for publication.

White, R. W. (1959). Motivation reconsidered: The concept of competence. *Psychological Review, 66,* 297–333.

Wiesenfeld, A., & Malatesta, C. Z. (1983). Assessing caregiver sensitivity to infants. In L. Rosenblum & H. Moltz (Eds.), *Symbiosis in parent–offspring.* NY: Plenum.

Wolfe, D.A. (1985). Child abusive parents: An empirical review and analysis. *Psychological Bulletin, 97,* 462–482.

Wolfe, D.A. (1987). *Child abuse: Implications for child development and psychopathology.* Newbury Park, CA: Sage.

Wolfe, D. A. (1988). Child abuse and neglect. In E. J. Mash & L. G. Terdal (Eds.), *Behavioral assessment of childhood disorders* (2nd ed., pp. 627–669). New York: Guilford Press.

Wolfe, D. A. (1990). Preventing child abuse means enhancing family functioning. *Canada's Mental Health, 38,* 27–29.

Wolfe, D.A. (in press). Child abuse intervention research: Implications for policy. In D. Cicchetti & S. Toth (Eds.), *Child abuse, child development, and social policy.* Norwood, NJ: Ablex.

Wolfe, D. A., & Bourdeau, P. A. (1987). Current issues in the assessment of abusive and neglectful parent–child relationships. *Behavioral Assessment, 9,* 271–290.

Wolfe, D. A., Edwards, B., Manion, I., & Koverola, C. (1988). Early intervention for parents at-risk for child abuse and neglect: A preliminary investigation. *Journal of Consulting and Clinical Psychology*, 56, 40–47.

Wolfe, D.A., Fairbank, J., Kelly, J.A., & Bradlyn, A.S. (1983). Child abusive parents' physiological responses to stressful and nonstressful behavior in children. *Behavioral Assessment, 5*, 363–371.

Wolfe, D.A., Kaufman, K., Aragona, J., & Sandler, J. (1981). *The child management program for abusive parents*. Winter Park, FL: Anna.

Wolfe, D.A., & Manion, I.G. (1984). Impediments to child abuse prevention: Issues and directions. *Advances in Behaviour Research and Therapy, 6*, 47–62.

Wolfe, D.A., & McGee, R. (1990). *Post traumatic stress and coping reactions: An interview scale for older children and adolescents*. Unpublished manuscript, University of Western Ontario.

Wolfe, D. A., & McGee, R.H. (1991). Assessment of children's emotional status. In R. Starr & D. Wolfe (Eds.), *The effects of child abuse and neglect: Issues and research* (pp. 257–277). NY: Guilford Press.

Wolfe, D.A., & Mosk, M.D. (1983). Behavioral comparisons of children from abusive and distressed families. *Journal of Consulting and Clinical Psychology, 51*, 702–708.

Wolfe, D. A., & Sandler, J. (1981). Training abusive parents in effective child management. *Behavior Modification, 5*, 320–335.

Wolfe, D.A., Sandler, J., & Kaufman, K. (1981). A competency-based parent training program for abusive parents. *Journal of Consulting and Clinical Psychology, 49*, 633–640.

Wolfe, D. A., Sas, L., & Wekerle, C. (1990, August). *Post-traumatic stress disorder symptoms among sexually abused children testifying before the court*. In P.A. Saigh (Chair), *International perspectives on post-traumatic stress disorder (PTSD)*. Symposium conducted at the annual convention of the American Psychological Association, Boston.

Wolfe, D. A., St. Lawrence, J., Graves, K., Brehony, K., Bradlyn, A., & Kelly, J. A. (1982). Intensive behavioral parent training for a child abusive mother. *Behavior Therapy, 13*, 438–451.

Wolfe, D. A., Wekerle, C., & McGee, R. (in press). Developmental disparities among abused children. In R.D. Peters & R. McMahon (Eds.), *Violence across the lifespan*. Newbury Park, CA: Sage.

Wright, L. (1976). The "sick but slick" syndrome as a personality component of parents of battered children. *Journal of Clinical Psychology, 32*, 41–45.

Wulrbert, M., Inglis, S., & Kriegsmann, E. (1975). Language delay and associated mother–child interactions. *Developmental Psychology, 2*, 61–70.

Zuravin, S.J. (1991). Suggestions for operationally defining child physical abuse and physical neglect. In R.H. Starr & D.A. Wolfe (Eds.), *The effects of child abuse and neglect: Issues and research* (pp. 100–128). NY: Guilford Press.

Index